Kate Llewellyn-Waters

the immunity cookbook

How to strengthen your immune system and boost long-term health, with 100 easy recipes

With a foreword by Dr Harriet Baker

Photography by Steven Joyce

Hardie Grant

QUADRILLE

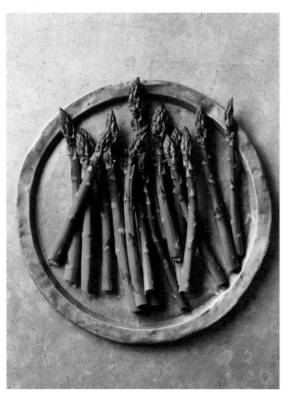

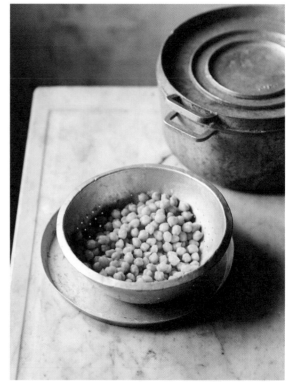

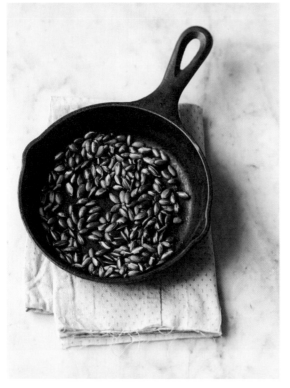

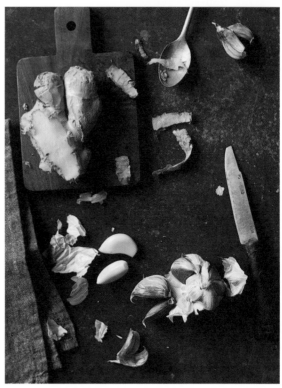

contents

foreword

As a medical doctor with a background in acute internal medicine and Medical Oncology, I have seen frequently how diet and lifestyle choices significantly affect the morbidity and mortality of my patients. The complex relationship between disease and inflammation is universally acknowledged. My particular interest is in the role of the immune system in fighting cancer, and this concept has been utilized in novel cancer immunotherapy, which uses the body's own immune system to fight the disease. Immunotherapy has improved outcomes in many types of cancer including lung cancer and melanoma. In addition, there is a growing body of evidence towards how cancer immunotherapy is even more effective when patients have an optimized gut microbiome.

Both the gut and immune system are highly complex systems, which as we now know, are intricately intertwined. Yet we hardly ever appreciate our crucial defence system until things go wrong. As the book highlights, when our immune systems aren't working as well as they should, we are more at risk of infectious disease, autoimmune conditions and allergies, as well as diseases such as cancer. Our immunity is closely associated with every area of our physical, emotional and mental wellbeing – it is the basis of our health. However, our fast-paced modern lives, chronic stress, poor nutrition habits, lack of physical activity, pollution and toxins threaten both our gut health and immunity.

The Immunity Cookbook is an evidence-based cookbook and reference guide detailing how our modern lives and ever-changing environment influence our gut health and immunity. As Kate shows, we need to balance our immune systems, and this, as is demonstrated, can be achieved with the appropriate nutrition choices, and by addressing areas such as gut health, exercise, stress management, mental health, sleep and sunlight exposure. Kate has drawn on scientific research in addition to alternative health literature to provide a detailed, balanced and informative reference guide, packed with 100 quick and straightforward breakfast, lunch, dinner and 'sweet treat' recipes that the whole family can enjoy. The book even includes a section on how to make certain 'homemade staples', which is very helpful. Kate employs a great balance of science, practical and effective strategies, anecdotes and delicious recipes. Additionally, all the advice is presented in a helpful reference table, which will make a significant difference to your health and everyday life. What excites me about this book is that instead of focusing on food exclusion, it is about enjoyable eating and living. It is not meant to be a quick fix, but if you can master the basics you can achieve the optimum from your gut health and immunity.

The Immunity Cookbook will provide you with the knowledge to make healthier choices, allowing you to achieve both improved gut health and stronger, balanced immunity. This book will change your current mindset about gut health and immunity, and has the potential to change your life forever, resulting in a healthier and happier you.

Dr Harriet Baker BSc MSc MBBS MRCP

introduction

My obsession with the digestive system began nearly 30 years ago, when I was a teenager and had to have an endoscopy to investigate a suspected hiatus hernia in my stomach. Being awake during this procedure, and watching, on screen, my upper gastrointestinal tract being explored, I decided there and then I wanted to learn as much as I could about this incredible system.

The gut is a fascinating organ, and as scientific research shows, the health of our gut plays a central role in our immunity, since an astonishing 70 per cent of our immune cells live in the gut. It is also home to trillions of microbes (different types of microorganisms such as bacteria, viruses and fungi), which make up the human microbiome. In fact, the gut microbiome is now regarded as an organ in its own right, often referred to as the 'second brain'. When we talk about the 'gut microbiome' we are referring to the microbes as well as their genetic material. These incredible microbes play a significant role in numerous areas of our health, and the activities of the microbiome are involved in most, if not all, of the human biological processes.

Our microbes live off the food we eat, so to thank us for feeding them, they provide lots of crucial services for our bodies, including:

- Producing key molecules, which strengthen the gut barrier and impact gut function

- Strengthening and balancing our immune system

- Regulating body weight by determining how much energy our body extracts from the food we eat, controlling hunger cues, and deciding how much our blood sugar is raised after a meal

- Communicating with other organs, such as our brain, heart and liver

- Making vitamins, amino acids, hormones and enzymes

- Metabolizing medications and deactivating toxins.

At present, we are in the midst of a worldwide immunity crisis, and never has it been a more appropriate time to address our immunity and gut health. Over millions of years our gut microbes, which make up our magical microbiome, have altered along with us, feeding off the food we eat. However, due to a nutrient-deficient and often inadequate diet, as well as antibiotic use, many of the gut microbes that evolved with us over millions of years no longer exist, or are present in much reduced quantities. The loss of these beneficial microbes influence our immunity, so it doesn't function as well as it ought. Luckily, through the power of nutrition and lifestyle choices, we have the ability to control and re-establish these missing microbes, helping them thrive, so that they can help us fight infections, balance an overactive immune system, and reduce our risk of allergies. To do this, we need to focus on eating a diet rich in evidence-based nutrients and foods, which promote the diversity of our gut bacteria species. This will allow the beneficial bacteria to thrive and also, encourage a strong, healthy gut lining. And, in turn, this will help us build strong and balanced immune systems, protecting us from infectious diseases, autoimmune diseases and allergies – all of which are, currently, at alarming levels in the Western world.

Fortunately, food choice is one of the most significant and valuable opportunities that we can embrace to improve our immunity and our gut health.

How the book works

My aim in writing this book is to provide you with an easy-to-follow guide, giving you the tools to help you make informed choices as to how to eat and live, so that you can achieve optimal gut health and healthy, balanced immunity.

The book provides an insight into your gut and immune system – how both systems work, how to look after them both, and what you can do to support your gut health and immune system in the long-term. I discuss the most effective and scientifically proven strategies as to how you can improve these areas, and have created 100 easy-to-make recipes, which will help you achieve optimal gut health and immunity.

Part 1 of the book explores how our extraordinary immune system and gut work, and also what autoimmune conditions and allergies are.

Part 2 discusses the most effective and evidence-based strategies to achieve better immunity. I explain how we can strengthen our gut health and immunity not only through diet, but also by addressing factors such as, exercise, sleep, mental health and sunlight. Part 3, which is the main and final part of the book, consists of 100 easy and quick recipes. Each of these recipes contains nutrients that have been demonstrated in scientific studies to benefit gut health and provide immune system support. All of the recipes use accessible ingredients, and I also offer gluten-free, dairy-free and vegan options to suit your requirements.

Furthermore, to help you get started on your gut health and immunity journey, I have also included two practical meal plans, and a go-to action plan (page 60), which summarizes all the guidance set out in the book in a simple table. This is a straightforward guide to help you begin to implement the discussed nutrition and lifestyle changes. By making the right nutrition choices, exercising appropriately, managing stress and ensuring optimal sleep and sufficient sunshine exposure, we can achieve strong and balanced gut health and immunity.

It's time to get started.

part 1:
the immune system

chapter 1:
hope in a time of crisis

> IMMUNITY means 'protection
> or exemption from something'.

There is no tissue or organ with a more significant influence on our health than the immune system. It is our body's defence system, and its main function is to distinguish self from non-self, identifying and defending our body from invaders such as bacteria, viruses, fungi, parasites and other pathogens. As well as fighting infection, our immune system has many other crucial functions, such as regulating body weight and metabolism, aiding the healing process, and even determining how we age. It is not located in one set of organized tissues, but is spread systematically throughout our body, consisting of many different cells, organs, and tissues that work together to fight infection, cellular damage and disease. Unfortunately, the immune system can, at times, make a mistake and attack itself, resulting in autoimmune disorders. For the immune system and its relevant tissues to be healthy, they must have adequate and optimal nutrition. Furthermore, undernourished individuals have a greater risk of adverse immune response and, irrespective of how mild a response, all immune responses place greater nutritional demands on the individual.

We are on the verge of a global immunity crisis – there has never been a more appropriate time to address our immunity, and how we can support it to promote optimal health. *The Immunity Cookbook* provides timely advice, supported by evidence-based research, and its aim is to give you the knowledge and practical guidance needed to help you balance and support your immune system.

To live a healthy and happy life we need as strong and balanced immunity as possible, which can be achieved by focusing on adopting a nutrient-dense and balanced diet, exercising appropriately, ensuring sufficient sleep, and managing stress effectively. First, let's take a closer look at the biggest threats to our immunity: infectious diseases, autoimmunity and allergies.

The threat is increasing

Every single day of our lives we are threatened with countless possible infectious risks, which our immune system often handles without us even realizing. Over the last twenty years we have experienced several devastating epidemics and pandemics, such as Covid-19, MERS (2012), H1N1 – also known as swine flu (2009), and SARS (2002). Out of all the infectious diseases of the last twenty years, at the time of writing swine flu has inflicted the most devastation, with the virus infecting as many as 1.4 billion people and killing between 151,700 and 575,400 worldwide. The 2009 swine flu pandemic was the second H1N1 pandemic the world had seen – the first being the 1918 Spanish flu, the most deadly pandemic in history, which killed more than 50 million individuals. We are now in the midst of another devastating pandemic, with more than 216 countries affected by Covid-19.

In addition to the public health threat that infectious diseases pose, autoimmune disorders are currently at near-epidemic levels, with more than 80 autoimmune disorders known at present. These disorders can cause extreme pain, everyday difficulties, and often put people at risk of premature death. Some of the most common autoimmune diseases include Type 1 diabetes, rheumatoid arthritis (RA) and systemic lupus (SLE). Four million people in the UK are living with an autoimmune condition. In the US, autoimmune disease is the third most common category of disease after cancer and cardiovascular disease, affecting 14.7 to 23.5 million people, which is equivalent 5 to 8 per cent of the population.

Allergies, like autoimmune diseases, are the result of the immune system overreacting. They now affect more than 20 per cent of the populations of most developed countries, and more than 150 million people in Europe suffer from chronic allergic diseases. The current prediction is that by 2025 half of the entire EU population will be affected. Globally, the World Allergy Organization (WAO) estimates allergy prevalence of the whole population by country ranges between 10 and 40 per cent, while in the UK allergies are believed to affect more than 1 in 4 people at some stage during their lives. They are especially common in children and, although some allergies disappear as a child gets older, many are permanent and will last a lifetime.

Let's take a closer look at some of the recent statistics:

- In 2016, the World Health Organization (WHO) stated that three infectious diseases were ranked in the top ten causes of death worldwide: lower respiratory infections (3 million deaths), diarrhoeal diseases (1.4 million deaths), and tuberculosis (1.3 million deaths).

- In the UK, an estimated 2 million people are living with a diagnosed food allergy.

- In the 20 years to 2012, there was a 615 per cent rise in the number of hospital admissions for anaphylaxis in the UK.

- In 2015, seven times as many people in Europe were admitted to hospital with severe allergic reactions than in 2005.

- The WHO estimates that 300 million individuals have asthma worldwide, and that with the current increasing rate this will grow to 400 million by 2025.

- In 2016, there were approximately 417,918 deaths from asthma, globally, according to WHO estimates.

- In the UK, 5.4 million individuals currently receive treatment for asthma. Of that, 1.1 million are children (1 in 11) and 4.3 million are adults (1 in 12).

- The WHO defines allergic rhinitis (hay fever) as one of the major chronic respiratory diseases globally. Allergic rhinitis is the most common type of non-infectious rhinitis, with between 10 and 30 per cent of all adults affected and almost 40 per cent of children[9].

The germ is nothing, the terrain is everything

In 1865, Louis Pasteur, along with Robert Koch, proposed Germ Theory, which stated that microorganisms invade a healthy body and subsequently result in disease. He also hypothesized that each germ produces one disease; thus, by eliminating that germ, the disease would also be eliminated. However, his contemporary, Claude Bernard, who worked with him to develop the process of 'pasteurization', believed that the state of the body, rather than an invading organism was the most important factor in disease. He hypothesized that if the body were healthy, the organism would not be able to invade, and there would be no ensuing disease. Pasteur, on his deathbed, admitted his former colleague's hypothesis was correct, and that 'the germ is nothing, the terrain is everything'. It is now very clear that not all diseases are caused by germs, as we can see, for example, with allergies.

The most powerful tool

The search is on for new forms of prevention and treatment to combat new diseases such as Covid-19. But what can we do to be protected against such debilitating diseases? Fortunately, one of the most powerful tools to which we all have access – and which is within our control – is our own immune system. It is our most valuable resource and our principal line of defence.

Our immune system is truly incredible and, for much of the time, it is protecting us against potentially harmful invaders without us even being aware. Through improved gut health, and nutritional and lifestyle modifications, our immunity can be supported to fight infection and disease. This is incredibly important, because as we age, the less effective our immune systems become.

Why we need to support our immunity

1. It defends our body against bacteria, viruses and fungi, which cause illness and disease.

2. Our immune function decreases as we age.

3. It can determine how quickly we age.

4. With one in two people predicted to get cancer at some point in their lives, a strong immune system is vital, as it has the ability to destroy cancer cells.

5. It eliminates all the toxins and chemicals that we have been exposed to over the course of a day, and also protects against radiation.

6. It helps to prevent auto-immune diseases and allergies.

Immunity suppressors

Immunity is essential to good health, from the moment of conception, when the mother's immune system begins to protect the developing baby, right through until old age. However, we are living in fast-paced times, and every day we are exposed to numerous factors that can suppress our immune systems, including:

- Obesity or malnutrition

- Incorrect balance of macro- and micronutrients

- Lack of, or excessive exercise

- Stress

- Sleep deprivation

- Insufficient exposure to sunlight

- Chemicals, such as food additives

- Pesticides and environmental toxins

- Air pollution

- Smoking

- Drugs and medications

It is imperative that we try to limit as many of the immunity suppressors as possible to ensure that our immune system remains balanced.

chapter 2: how the immune system works

An overview of the immune system

The immune system is the body's biological defence system, consisting of many different cells, organs and tissues that work together patrolling every component of the body, defending against invaders and cellular damage. Let's take a closer look at this wonderful system, which is protecting us every single day of our lives.

The lymphatic system

The lymphatic system is a drainage system that helps to get rid of waste and toxins. It runs throughout the whole body as a conduit for the fluid known as lymph. Lymph carries out one of the most important jobs in our immunity – surveillance, a vital daily immune-cell job. Our white blood cells, which we will look at in detail later in this chapter, use the lymph to patrol all corners of the body, 'surveilling' for infection.

The system is made up of lymphatic vessels that connect to lymph nodes (small kidney-bean-shaped organs) that filter the lymph. The vessels themselves are tube-shaped, like our blood vessels, and transport the lymph, which eventually enters the blood circulation. Unlike blood, lymphatic fluid is not pumped, but squeezed through the vessels when we use our muscles, which is why exercise is so crucial to our health. If our lymph is supported by movement, regular physical activity is key to ensuring a healthy lymphatic system, and ultimately strong immunity. The one-way valves in the lymph vessels keep the lymph moving, and prevent it from flowing backwards. The lymph gradually drains in the direction of the large lymphatic ducts, and it is at this point the lymph (now filtered) returns to the blood in the veins.

Five facts about the lymphatic system
1. The lymphatic system plays a crucial role in our immunity.

2. It plays a key role in fluid balance, and the absorption of fats and immunity-nourishing fat-soluble vitamins A, D, E and K.

3. The lymph nodes swell in response to infection, which is when they may feel enlarged under your skin. Check the glands at the side of your neck, groin, or under your armpits next time you have an infection.

4. If lymph nodes remain swollen, and if you have other symptoms, you should see a medical practitioner.

5. Insufficient digestion and an imbalanced gut microbiome can also affect the lymphatic system.

The lymph nodes

The lymph nodes are small bean-shaped organs that store immune cells, and it is in these nodes that our immune cells inspect for bacteria, viruses, fungi or other pathogens. In the human body, there are approximately 500–600 lymph nodes. When we have an infection, they become swollen because of the accumulation of bacteria, immune cells and lymph. You can feel some lymph nodes where they are close to the surface of your skin, often on the sides of your neck or under your arms, and they are more prominent when we are experiencing an infection.

The thymus

The thymus gland is located behind the sternum (the breast bone) and is only active until puberty. However, it has a significant responsibility when it's active, such as helping the body defend itself against autoimmunity. Throughout childhood and even before birth, the thymus is highly active in the production and maturation of infection-fighting white blood cells, known as T-lymphocytes (T cells). In fact, it produces all your T cells, which are vital for strong immunity, by puberty. The thymus is truly unique, since it is at its maximum size in childhood. After puberty, it begins to shrink, so much so that by the age of 75 it is more or less just fatty tissue!

As well as playing a crucial role in the lymphatic system, the thymus is important in the endocrine system, which is the collection of glands that produce hormones that regulate metabolism, growth and development, tissue function, sexual function, reproduction, sleep and mood.

The spleen

This is an organ in the upper left-hand side of your abdomen that consists of lymph tissue. It has some important functions, including:

- destroying certain harmful 'invaders'

- regulating the level of blood cells (white blood cells, red blood cells and platelets)

- getting rid of any old/damaged red blood cells.

The spleen is an important part of your immune system, but you can survive without it, as the liver can take over many of its functions. The liver also produces lymph, and Kupffer cells, which neutralize bacteria, yeasts and toxins.

Bone marrow

Bone marrow is the tissue located inside your bones, which contains stem cells and is vital in producing the blood cells that are crucial to our immunity. After early childhood, most immune cells are produced from the bone marrow.

Red blood cells

At a very basic level, red blood cells simply capture 'invaders' and then pass them to the white blood cells to deal with.

White blood cells

These are the cells involved in our main immune defence, and are present in lymph as well as in blood. There are three main types of white blood cells – or leukocytes: granulocytes, monocytes and lymphocytes:

Lymphocytes

Lymphocytes are white blood cells which are highly capable of eliminating harmful 'invaders'. They are made in the bone marrow and found in the blood and lymph tissue. We have an incredible 2×10^{12} lymphocytes (approximately) in our body, making the immune system comparable in cell mass to the brain or liver. Two types of lymphocytes are B cells and T cells, which originate from stem cells in the bone marrow. From the bone marrow, some cells travel to the thymus, where they become T cells, while others remain where they are, becoming B cells.

The job of B cells is to make antibodies, which are proteins produced by the immune system to combat antigens. Every B cell produces a single species of antibody – each with a unique antigen-binding site[12].

> **AN ANTIGEN** is anything which provokes an antibody response. An allergy-provoking food can be an antigen.

> **ANTIBODY SPECIFICITY** – each individual antibody precisely identifies one specific antigen. So, for example, an antibody that identifies the measles virus cannot identify the mumps virus.

The role of the T cells is to control the immune response to foreign substances and help kill cancer cells. They do this by destroying cells in the body that have been taken over by viruses or become cancerous.

A third type of lymphocyte, known as a natural killer or NK cell, comes from the same place as B and T cells. NK cells respond quickly to several foreign substances and kill virus-infected cells and cancer cells.

There are different types of B cells and T cells that have specific roles in the body and the immune system.

Antibodies

In our plasma, we also have antibodies, which are proteins produced by the immune system that aid in defending against infection. They help to destroy harmful germs by quickly eliminating them or by preventing them from infecting cells. As we have seen earlier in the chapter, when we are challenged by foreign material (bacteria, viruses or other pathogens) the first response of certain immune cells, such as macrophages, is to engulf these invaders (antigens) and process them. This essentially creates a plan that is used for the development of an immune response that results in the production of antibodies. The unique feature of antibodies produced in response to an antigen is that they are synthesized in such a way that they are highly specific for that antigen. Thus, they can chemically interact and bind only with that particular antigen, neutralizing it, and/or aiding in its destruction and removal from the body.

There are five different classes of antibodies, also referred to as immunoglobulins (Igs): IgA, IgD, IgE, IgG and IgM. These antibodies differ in many ways, including in their overall structures, and they work by recognizing and sticking to specific proteins, such as those found on the surfaces of bacteria and viruses.

When the body meets a germ for the first time, immune cells produce antibodies that specifically recognize proteins associated with that particular germ. Once we have recovered from an infection or had a vaccine, some of these antibody-producing immune cells can remain in the body as memory cells, thus providing immunity against future infections with the same germ. Since memory cells and antibodies are already present, next time the body encounters the same germ, the immune response is much quicker and can stop the infection in its tracks.

Antibody tests can be helpful in determining whether or not someone already has immunity to a particular infection. However, they cannot detect if antibodies are present immediately, since it takes some time for the body to produce antibodies against a new germ.

Autoimmunity, allergies and antibodies

The National Institute of Allergy and Infectious Diseases (NIAID) in the US defines 'immune tolerance' as the prevention of an immune response against a certain antigen. While the immune system does not usually attack our own cells, when we do lose immune tolerance, allergies and autoimmune disorders can result. Simply put, antibodies that recognize the body's own proteins, instead of proteins from infectious germs can cause harm. In autoimmune conditions, such as rheumatoid arthritis, lupus and multiple sclerosis, an individual will generate antibodies that attach to their body's own proteins and attack healthy cells.

Allergies involve a class of antibodies called immunoglobulin E (IgE). When these antibodies detect allergens, they trigger immune cells to release histamine and other inflammatory molecules, which can cause the symptoms associated with allergic reactions.

Immunological memory

One of the most important characteristics of the immune response is its ability to recall past infections. This incredible memory protects you from being reinfected with a previous bug, while reducing the spread of infection in a community. Immunological memory can last for a very long time. In fact, a study reported that when the participants were assessed, their memory for the measles infection was declining so gradually, it would take in excess of 3,000 years to reduce by half[13]. These enduring changes are why, when we vaccinate, the protection provides mostly long-term benefits. The goal of vaccination is to induce long-lasting protective immune memory. Although most vaccines induce good memory responses, the type of memory induced by different vaccines may be considerably different. In addition, memory responses to the same vaccine have been shown to be influenced by age and environmental and genetic factors.

Immunological memory must be dispersed throughout the body. Circulating antibodies are transported in the blood, going everywhere the circulation does, therefore immunological memory also forms outside the bloodstream within tissues. With our attentive killer cells on guard where the immune defences broke down previously, they are poised ready to attack if reinfection threatens. Those cells now know how to combat the specific germ, which is the reason why, in the majority of cases, you only encounter some diseases, such as chickenpox, once.

> **IMMUNOLOGICAL MEMORY** is the ability of the immune system to respond more rapidly and effectively to pathogens that have been previously encountered.

Unfortunately, there are some devious viruses that have established ways to dodge our immunological memory, such as the rhinovirus, which is a cause of the common cold. The rhinovirus infection has also been associated with lower respiratory tract symptoms and it is widely acknowledged that it is also a significant cause of asthma severity in children. These sly viruses are so successful because they are continually altering the recognition code on their surfaces.

Genes and our immunity

Each person's immunity is unique and we know that it is influenced by numerous aspects, including genetics and environment. To explore the opposing influences of nature versus nurture, researchers at Stanford University, California, conducted a twin study. The trial included 210 healthy identical and fraternal twins, between 8 and 82 years old.

It posited that if a trait is hereditary, it will be more probable that identical twins will share it than fraternal twins. The participants had blood samples taken and 204 parameters of their immune systems were measured, including 95 kinds of immune cells and 51 kinds of proteins.

Researchers observed that 77 per cent of the 204 parameters measured were dominated by non-heritable, i.e. environmental, influences. In addition, younger twins were more alike than older twins, indicating that as the twins advanced in years and were exposed to different environments, over time their immune systems also changed.

Furthermore, genetic influence in response to the flu vaccine was also evaluated. We know that some individuals can react more strongly to vaccines than others, producing more antibodies. Thus, if this trait were genetic, identical twins should have responses that were alike. However, the responses to the seasonal influenza vaccination were also determined largely by non-heritable factors, most likely due to repeated exposure to different strains.

These findings highlighted the adaptive nature of the immune system, and that as we age our immune systems change in increasingly individualized and unique ways. Even twins who are identical, appear to have immune systems that become dissimilar as they mature, influenced by each twin making thousands of individual nutrition and lifestyle choices, and responses to their environment.

Ageing and our immunity

Ageing is associated with a progressive decline of the immune system, commonly referred to as 'immunosenescence'. There are several consequences of age-dependent immunosenescence, including increased risk of infection and autoimmune diseases, reduced response to vaccination, and chronic inflammation.

The exact mechanisms involved in immunosenescence are not fully understood, but one of the most significant causes is the regression and shrinking of the thymus. After puberty, our thymus gland begins to gradually shrink. In time, it will be little more than fatty tissue, losing the ability to produce new T cells. Thus, elderly individuals are potentially not as able to respond to immune challenges as robustly as someone younger.

Another aspect of ageing is inflammation, which involves progressively increased levels of chronic inflammation known as 'inflammageing'. It is believed to accelerate the process of biological ageing and to worsen many age-related diseases.

When it comes to ageing immunity, it certainly does not mean your health has to decline as you age. There are several areas of our lives that we can address to ensure our immunity stays in balance and these are explored in Part 2.

chapter 3:
infectious diseases, autoimmune conditions and allergies

'The constancy of the internal environment is the condition for a free and independent life.'

Claude Bernard, French physiologist

The human immune system is undeniably highly complex, and our precious immunity is threatened every day by suppressors, including inadequate nutrition, inappropriate levels of exercise, chronic stress, air pollution, lack of sunlight and environmental toxins. Left to decline and weaken, it can go haywire, resulting in us being more susceptible to infections, allergies and autoimmune diseases. This chapter takes a look at what can happen when things get out of control.

Infectious diseases

Until the end of the twentieth century, infectious diseases were responsible for the greatest global burden of premature death. Over the last 500 years, worldwide pandemics of infectious diseases, such as influenza, cholera and smallpox placed whole populations in danger of being completely wiped out. However, in high-income countries, improved sanitation and living conditions began to reduce the toll of infectious disease, and by the mid-twentieth century vaccines and the accessibility to antibiotics decreased the burden of infectious diseases even further.

Bacteria, along with viruses, are the most common source of infectious diseases, with antibiotics often used to combat bacterial infection. However, emerging pandemic viral infections are a continual threat, and while antibiotics can treat bacterial infections, comparatively few antiviral drugs have been developed to treat these emerging viral infections. Our first line of defence against a viral infection is the interferon system. Interferons are cytokines, and they're named for their ability to 'interfere' with viral replication by protecting cells from virus infection. This system is designed to block the spread of virus infection in the body, and is highly dependent on adequate vitamin C and the mineral manganese. Unfortunately, some viral infections aren't able to be eliminated by the immune system, and the viruses hide in cells. These hidden viruses are able to be re-activated, which leads to repeated attacks, such as the recurring cold sores of the herpes virus.

Epidemics and pandemics have always had major social and economic impacts on affected populations, but in the modern world the impacts are truly global. Despite major advances in infectious disease research and treatment, the control and elimination of these diseases face significant challenges.

More men than women die of infectious disease

Fatality rates of infectious diseases are often higher in males than females. This has also been observed in data concerning Covid-19, where data from the Centers of Disease Control and Prevention indicated that, in England and Wales, men account for 60 per cent of all deaths and in Malaysia 78 per cent. According to findings from past respiratory disease studies, it could be due to the role that testosterone and oestrogen play. Alternatively, it may be due to the fact that the X chromosome (of which females have two, but males have only one), has more immune-related genes, thus providing females with stronger immunity to defend against certain infections, such as Covid-19. Generally, females tend to mount a stronger immune response, which helps them to clear infections quicker. However, while this more robust immune response helps to combat unwanted invaders, it does make women more susceptible to immune disorders.

Autoimmune conditions

Autoimmune disease occurs when the immune system mounts an attack against healthy tissue. In autoimmunity, the immune system recognizes, targets and causes damage to normal tissues, such as skin, kidneys, pancreas, the nervous system and the body's joints. There are over 80 autoimmune conditions, each affecting different parts of the body. For example, in Type 1 diabetes, the immune system destroys the cells that make insulin; in rheumatoid arthritis, the lining of the joints are attacked; and in multiple sclerosis, the coating around nerves is damaged.

While no exact figure exists in the UK for the total number of people affected by the 80 or more identified autoimmune disorders, it has been estimated that approximately four million people have an autoimmune condition – which is more than 6 per cent of the population. The US National Institutes of Health (NIH) estimates that approximately 23.5* million Americans live with an autoimmune disease and that its prevalence

is on the rise, while the American Autoimmune Related Diseases Association (AARDA) says that approximately 50 million Americans live with an autoimmune disease. (*The NIH only includes 24 diseases for which they had epidemiology studies they considered appropriate available.)

Furthermore, having one autoimmune condition makes developing another more likely, with up to a third of the four million people affected by autoimmunity living with more than one autoimmune condition[20]. This can result in extremely complicated and multifaceted health needs and, ultimately, makes everyday life significantly more difficult.

- According to Diabetes UK, there are around 400,000 people in the UK with Type 1 diabetes and this rate is growing at a rate of 3 per cent per annum. Whilst in the US approximately 1.6 million have Type 1 diabetes, including 187,000 children and adolescents (ADA, 2020).

- Rheumatoid arthritis (RA) affects roughly 700,000 people in the UK, according to the British Society for Rheumatology. RA also affects over 1.3 million Americans (Rheumatology Org, 2020).

- At least 115,000 people in the UK live with Crohn's disease. Whilst in the US, around 780,000 people are currently living with this debilitating disease (Crohn's Colitis Foundation, 2020).

- A 2014 study estimated a UK-wide figure of 127,000 for prevalence of MS, with the number of people affected by the condition growing at a rate of 2.4 per cent per year. And, nearly 1 million American adults have been diagnosed with MS (National MS Society, 2020).

- Lupus is thought to affect up to 50,000 people in the UK. The Lupus Foundation of America, believes that approximately 1.5 million Americans, and 5 million people worldwide have a form of lupus (Roper, 2012).

Disturbingly, autoimmune conditions are on the rise, with treatments to manage them already costing billions. Unfortunately, they are poorly understood. Research has indicated that genetic predisposition explains approximately 30 per cent of all autoimmune disorders, while 70 per cent are owing to environmental factors, including dietary issues, gut dysbiosis (see page 27), infections, and exposure to toxic chemicals[21]. As we know, in general, women tend to have a stronger immune response, which helps to clear infections quickly, but it also increases vulnerability to immune disorders[18]. In the United States alone, women represent 80 per cent of all cases of autoimmune disease.

While it is evident that genetics play a role in autoimmunity, we still don't know exactly how genes are involved. Having a family member with lupus, for example, does increase your risk of also getting lupus, but some families have several family members who all have different autoimmune disorders. Additionally, it appears there are lots of genes involved in the immune response on the X chromosome, and because, as we saw earlier, women have two X chromosomes while men have only one, women have more of those immune genes. Genetics alone isn't enough to cause autoimmune disease. Professor Johann E. Gudjonsson of the University of Michigan discovered that females have more of a molecular switch called VGLL3 in their skin than males, and that more of this VGLL3 may be what provokes an increased immune response in females.

Nearly 50 per cent of women who develop an autoimmune disease do so in the first year after pregnancy. Then, as a woman enters menopause, the reduction in female sex hormones leads to a considerable decrease in immune function, leaving it similar to, or even less capable than that of a male[22]. This can be a period when autoimmunity symptoms improve or, due to a reduction in immune function, symptoms may worsen. Thus, as we get older, we need to focus on supporting our immunity more than ever.

While we know that certain genes or being exposed to certain environmental factors can make some autoimmune conditions more likely, that's not the whole picture – something is going wrong with the immune system, and we don't fully know why, as yet. Currently, autoimmune conditions cannot be cured, which means that for many people who develop an autoimmune disease, a lifetime of daily management and potential health complications lies ahead.

Allergies

Like autoimmune conditions, incidence of allergies is increasing. In fact, allergy is the most common chronic disease in Europe, with up to 20 per cent of patients affected by an allergy living with an incapacitating or life-threatening form, and fighting daily with the anxiety and distress of a potential asthma attack, anaphylaxis, or even death[23]. In addition, more than 50 million Americans have experienced various types of allergies each year, and up to 2 million, or 8 per cent, of children in the US are estimated to be affected by food allergies[24].

Similarly to autoimmune disease, allergy is caused by an inappropriate immune response, and results when the body alters its normal immune response to an offending allergen (a substance that provokes an antibody response). An allergic response can be a result of a variety of different stimuli, such as pollen, medications (such as the antibiotic penicillin), or a particular food. Allergic responses are very specific because they are adaptive immune responses. Thus, a hay fever sufferer's condition is caused by one type of pollen, not just by any pollen, and a patient with an allergy to penicillin may be safe taking other kinds of antibiotic. While in the instance of contact allergies, such as sensitivity to nickel or washing detergents, it is the lymphocytes and macrophages that over-react, in most other allergies it is the antibody response that is over-reactive.

Allergies are the most common type of acquired immune disease, and they usually depend on an IgE-mediated immune response to the antigen.

IgE antibodies attach themselves to 'mast cells' and, when the allergen combines with its specific IgE antibody, the IgE molecule triggers the mast cell to release granules containing histamine and other chemicals that cause the symptoms of allergy, such as asthma, eczema, hay fever and hives.

The reasons for the rising rate in allergies are not fully understood, but we do know that genetics plays a role, since allergies have a tendency to run in families. Another theory is that it may be the result of living in a cleaner, more sterile and germ-free environment, which decreases the number of germs our immune systems have to deal with. It is thought this may cause our immune system to then over-react when it comes into contact with harmless substances. The 'hygiene hypothesis' proposes that modern standards of public health, which have had a significant effect on the timing and type of infections that children encounter as they grow up, have altered the balance of the immune response. On a positive note, childhood mortality is considerably reduced due to improved public health, but on the other hand, immune systems, which develop in this sterile world may be less 'educated', and potentially more inclined to make a mistake. Such hypotheses are very tricky to prove, but various findings have confirmed the intricate and highly complex relationship that exists between the immune system and the environment.

Atopic conditions

Atopic diseases tend to occur in a progression, termed the 'atopic march', which refers to the natural history of allergic diseases as they develop over the course of infancy and childhood. The initial manifestation of atopic disease in infancy or early childhood is often eczema, followed by the staggered development of food allergy, hay fever and asthma.

ATOPHY or BEING ATOPIC means having a genetic tendency for your immune system to make increased levels of IgE antibodies to certain allergens. An atopic individual is likely to have more than one allergic condition during their lifetime, such as eczema, asthma, hay fever or food allergy.

Contact with an allergen can bring about various forms of eczema and involves an over-active response by the immune system. While the exact cause of developing an atopic condition like eczema is unknown, it is not down to one single thing, and often food allergies can play a part, as may inadequate food choices, obesity, exposure to stress, air pollution, infections, antibiotics and vitamin D deficiency. Further, research has shown that vitamin D has confirmed effects on immunity, which may be significant in the progression, severity and course of eczema, asthma and food allergies. Deficiency in vitamin D is a global issue, which could be a reason why there has been a keen rise in allergic diseases that have resulted over the last sixty years.

Food allergies

Food allergies are on the rise, and some of the most common offenders include foods such as cow's milk, egg, peanuts, tree nuts, soy, wheat, shellfish and fish. A true food allergy causes an immune-system reaction involving IgE antibodies, which affects numerous organs in the body, causing a range of symptoms, such as hives, digestive upsets, swelling in the face or throat or itching. In some cases, an allergic food reaction can be life-threatening, resulting in anaphylaxis. If you have an immediate reaction after eating a food, it is most likely to be an allergic response. In contrast, food intolerance symptoms can result fairly quickly, but are often delayed by up to 48 hours and last for hours or even days. They are also generally less serious and often limited to digestive issues.

Food allergy facts
- It is estimated that between 1 and 10 per cent of adults and children have a food hypersensitivity. However, as many as 20 per cent of the population experience some reaction to foods that make them think they have a food hypersensitivity.

- Around 11–26 million members of the European population are estimated to suffer from food allergy. If this prevalence is projected onto the world's population of 7 billion, it converts into 240–550 million individuals with potential food allergies[9].

- Food allergy tends to affect approximately 3–6 per cent of children in the developed world. However, in the UK, it is estimated that the prevalence for food allergy is 7.1 per cent in breast-fed infants, with 1 in 40 developing peanut allergy and 1 in 20 developing egg allergy.

Correct diagnosis of a food allergy is crucial to identify individuals who could have critical and deadly allergic reactions, and also to eliminate potential allergies that may result in avoidable dietary restrictions. Medically supervised oral food challenges (OFC) remain the most definitive test in the diagnosis of food allergy, with the majority of oral food challenges being carried out openly, so the individual and medical professional conducting the challenge are aware of what food is being tested. However, OFCs that are blinded can follow two different forms:

single-blinded is when the individual may not know what they are eating; and a double-blind OFC is when both the medical professional and patient are unaware if it is a 'placebo' or 'test food' that is being eaten. (If testing a potential allergy for soy, and soy is hidden in a cracker – this is a test food. Another cracker that tastes and looks just the same, but without the soy, is the placebo.) The American Academy of Allergy, Asthma and Immunology (AAAAI) considers the double-blind oral food challenge as the best test, as it reduces potential anxiety-associated reactions. However, blinded challenges are seldom conducted in clinical practices, and are generally performed in research studies. If a subject is found to have a true food allergy, treatment is usually complete exclusion of that food.

Food intolerances

As we have seen, it is the immune response that determines whether an individual may have a true food allergy. Where the immune system causes the reaction in food allergy, it is the digestive system that triggers the reaction in a food intolerance. This is when your body can't properly break a substance down, or your body reacts to a food you're sensitive to; for example, lactose intolerance is when your body can't break down lactose – a sugar found in dairy products. Symptoms of food intolerance may include gas, bloating, diarrhoea, constipation, digestive cramping and nausea. There are lots of reasons why you may experience a food intolerance:

- lacking the digestive enzyme you need to break down a particular food

- reacting adversely to substances added to food, such as additives and preservatives

- a chemical sensitivity reaction to food components, such as caffeine

- sensitivity to naturally occurring dietary components, such as fructans (found in artichokes, cabbage and leeks), that may cause IBS symptoms.

Keeping a food diary can be useful in helping you narrow down food intolerances. If you still can't pinpoint the culprit, you may wish to try an elimination diet (see page 31). This strategy involves removing foods that are most commonly associated with intolerances for about two weeks, at which point foods are then re-introduced, one at a time. You may wish to undertake a guided elimination diet with the support of a nutritionist or dietician who can advise you, thus avoiding any potential nutrient deficiencies.

Allergies are especially common in children, with some disappearing as the child gets older; however, many are lifelong. Adults can also develop allergies to things they weren't previously allergic to, which is exactly what happened to me in 2015.

My story

I have had numerous operations in my life, but only twice in 43 years have I been bedridden by an illness. The first was when I contracted the Epstein-Barr virus (EBV), which is responsible for glandular fever, at the age of 15.

The second time occurred in 2015, shortly after the birth of my second child. I had been working hard the months before I got ill, but what started as a minor cold developed into viral chest pneumonia, which left me bedridden for two weeks. That was bad enough, but it was what I developed immediately afterwards that completely derailed me.

It was a cold December day, and I remember being delighted that I was well enough to go outside for a walk with my 12-week-old son. However, after less than two minutes outside, I felt as though I was burning and itching all over, but especially in my face. My face was inflamed and covered in red and white patches, as if I had been wearing a ski-mask. I also had welts all over my body. At that stage, I knew I had had an allergic reaction, and went through what I had eaten or drank prior to going outside, but there was nothing out of the ordinary. After about an

hour, the welts and swelling started to subside. Unfortunately, it happened the next day, and the next… I dreaded going out. Even for the daily drop-off and pick-up, I would take an anti-histamine prior to leaving the house. This didn't reduce the burning, swelling and itching, so I booked in to see my GP. It emerged that I had 'cold urticaria', which affects about 0.05 per cent of the population.

The cause of most cases of cold urticaria is unknown, but it is thought in some cases to be triggered by an infectious disease, an insect bite, certain medications or blood cancers. My doctor advised that the allergy could last for a minimum of five years, and the only treatment available was a daily antihistamine, which didn't improve my symptoms at all.

I realized that the pressure of recently giving birth, of being mum to two children under three, working hard, and also writing up a substantial research paper had taken their toll and pushed my immune system to the limit. I believed I had contracted a minor virus that my body would normally have fought off with ease, but excess stress and severe lack of sleep meant that my immunity at that point was unable to fight it off.

Back to basics

During my son's birth, I had had a C-section and also underwent a two-hour bowel operation. Afterwards, I had been given antibiotics to prevent infection. It was therefore very likely that much of my 'good' bacteria had been wiped out. As we know, antibiotics can reduce gut bacteria diversity in just three days, with the effects of a short course lasting for years. In the days following the frantic activity of having a new-born and a longer-than-intended hospital stay, I hadn't thought about addressing my gut health. For 12 weeks following my son's birth, sleep had been non-existent, while my emotional and physical stress was the highest it had ever been. Therefore, I decided to go back to basics, and followed exactly the same programme I outline in Chapter 5 (page 31). After six weeks, my allergy had gone.

chapter 4:
all disease begins in the gut

> 'All disease begins in the gut.'
>
> Hippocrates, c.460–370BC

Existing research shows that there is a significant amount of interaction between the body's immune system and bacteria in the gut. Our many physiological systems in the body work in synergy together, and our gut microbiome and immune system are very much connected, especially when you consider the fact that approximately 70–80 per cent of your immune system is in your gut. Our microbiome and immunity are certainly not independent of each other, but appear to have an extremely close and important connection.

The microbiome

The human microbiome, which is now known as an organ in its own right and often referred to as the 'second brain', is composed of communities of bacteria, viruses and fungi, the majority of which live in our guts. An estimated 100 trillion microbes, weighing over four pounds, exist in the guts alone. When we define 'microbiome', we are referring to the microbes and their genetic material. Over millions of years, the microbes that comprise our microbiome have changed with us and live off the food we eat. Extraordinarily, the activities of the microbiome are involved in most, if not all, of the human biological processes. The microbes, to reward us for feeding them, provide lots of vital services to our bodies, such as extracting energy from our food, controlling the calories we absorb, providing enzymes, manufacturing vitamins, working with our

nervous system, producing numerous hormones, and influencing our immunity.

> MICROBES are types of microorganisms. The major groups of microorganisms are bacteria, archaea, fungi (yeasts and moulds), algae, protozoa and viruses.
>
> MICROBIOTA refers to all the microbes in a community, such as bacteria, viruses and fungi. It was first defined by Lederberg and McCray, who stressed the significance of microorganisms in the body and their role in human health.
>
> MICROBIOME refers to the microorganisms AND their genes.

Over the last ten years, it has become evident that the gut microbiome plays an important role in shaping the immune system, as well as contributing to health and disease. Our understanding of the gut microbiome is also increasing quickly, due to the development and application of technological advances, particularly genomic approaches. This is probably best demonstrated by large-scale studies, including the Human Microbiome Project, which was performed over ten years and in two phases. This was a United States NIH research initiative, to improve understanding of the microbiota involved in health and disease. Furthermore, the Human Microbiome Project helped establish the extensiveness of microbial variation and function across large populations, in addition to determining associations between microbiota alterations and disease states.

The role of the microbiota in regulating metabolic activity has been demonstrated with increasing evidence, indicating an involvement in glucose regulation, weight management and also regulation of the hypothalamic-pituitary-adrenal (HPA) axis. The autonomic nervous system, the HPA axis, and the nerves within the gastrointestinal tract connect the gut and the brain. This allows the brain to affect gut activities, such as the activity of immune effector cells. If the HPA axis is disrupted, not only does this wreak havoc on our microbiota but also our immunity.

Our gut microbes play a crucial role in educating, training and modulating our immunity, lending it a helping hand to distinguish friend from foe. Furthermore, some researchers believe that the increase in autoimmune disease may be the result of a disruption in the relationship between our bodies and the microbes that we evolved with. Unlike other endocrine organs, the microbiota has significant plasticity and can change considerably and quickly in response to diet[37].

> **PLASTICITY** is the adaptability of an organism to changes in its environment or differences between its various habitats.

While our wonderful microbes clearly impact us, we can also influence them. In fact, what we eat and how we live has a massive effect on the type of microbes that make up our microbiomes, as we will discover.

Main functions of our microbes include:

· Educating, training and supporting our immunity

· Producing important molecules that strengthen the gut barrier

· Feeding on fibre and antioxidants from plant-based foods

· Making vitamins, amino acids, hormones and chemical messengers

· Metabolizing medications and deactivating toxins

· Influencing gut movement and function

· Communicating with our brain, heart and liver

· Regulating body weight

Bacterial baptism

So, how do we get these marvellous microbes?

A recent large-scale study, the largest ever study of neonatal microbiomes, provided further understanding about the development of the microbiome and whether the birth delivery method played a role in this. The study analysed 1,679 gut bacteria samples from almost 600 healthy babies and 175 mothers. Stool samples were performed on babies at four, seven or twenty-one days old, who had been delivered vaginally or by Caesarean section (C-section). The researchers employed DNA sequencing and genomics analysis to study which bacteria were in the babies' guts. They reported a significant difference between the methods of delivery. Babies born by vaginal delivery had many more beneficial bacteria from their mothers than those that were delivered by C-section.

Previous limited studies had suggested that, while travelling down the birth canal, vaginal bacteria were swallowed by the baby, however this study reported that very few of the mother's vaginal bacteria were present in the babies' guts, with no difference observed between those delivered vaginally or by C-section. In fact, the researchers discovered it was the mother's gut bacteria that comprised much of the microbiome in the babies born vaginally. On the other hand, babies born via C-section had significantly fewer of these bacteria and instead had more bacteria associated with hospital environments present in their guts. It should be noted that women who have a C-section are given antibiotics before the procedure to limit the risk of post-operative infections, which means that the baby also receives antibiotics via the placenta. This could perhaps, in part, explain some of the microbiome differences reported between the vaginal and C-section births.

Some babies up to 12 months old were also followed up, and the researchers found the differences in gut bacteria between the babies delivered vaginally and those born by C-section had essentially evened out. The researchers confirmed that their findings demonstrated that as the babies age and 'ingest' bacteria from the food they eat and from their environment, the vaginally born and C-section-delivered babies' microbiomes become more alike. This is an exciting area of research. However, large follow-up studies are required to determine if the initial differences do influence health outcomes.

As a mother, I know that vaginal birth is not always possible. Both of my children were delivered by C-section due to the presence of fibroids. In many cases, a C-section is a life-saving procedure, and can be the best option for a woman and her baby. Experts from the Royal College of Obstetricians and Gynaecologists confirmed that these findings should not deter women from having a C-section birth. Also, if you do end up having a C-section birth, you are still able to encourage a healthy and balanced biome for your baby.

One of the best ways of doing this is by breast-feeding. Breast milk consists of carbohydrates, fat and protein, as well as sugars called oligosaccharides. While the baby can't digest these complex sugars, they do feed the 'good'

bacteria in the baby's gut and promote accurate development of its immunity. As baby grows up, his or her food choices broaden, which in turn influences the microbiome. When baby reaches toddlerhood, around the age of three, their microbiome will be more or less established. However, it can still be altered by nutrition, diet changes, antibiotic use and infections acquired.

- Babies that are breast-fed are half as likely to develop asthma or eczema as a baby who is exclusively bottle-fed.

- The gut microbiome is believed to be crucial for the development of the immune system.

- Lack of exposure to the 'right' microbes in early childhood has been associated with autoimmune diseases and allergies[39].

In conclusion, although we can't do anything about how we were born, or whether we were breast- or bottle-fed, we do have the power to choose what we subsequently eat and thereby feed our gut microbiomes.

The missing microbes

Our microbiota plays a fundamental role in the education, training and function of our immunity. Learning to recognize a threat – and what is not a threat – is key. It is believed that a rich and diverse microbiome allows the gut immune system to remain 'stimulated and in a constant state of readiness, so there will be no over-reaction to strange proteins'.[40]

We certainly don't want our immune system attacking our 'good' gut microbes, which are crucial to our health and well being. However, due to a highly processed and often nutrient-deficient diet, in addition to antibiotic use, many of the gut microbes that have evolved with us over millions of years are either no longer present or exist in much smaller quantities. This loss of these microbes impacts our immunity, so it doesn't perform and behave as well as it should. Fortunately, through our nutrition and lifestyle choices, we have the power to cultivate and re-establish these missing microbes, in order to successfully fight infection, bring an over-active immune system back into balance and decrease our risk of allergies.

The epigenetic link

It is generally acknowledged that factors such as diet, lifestyle and genetics have the greatest influence on shaping the gut microbiome. While we can't change our genes, we can influence the composition of the different species of bacteria in our guts through diet and lifestyle choices. Furthermore, researchers have found that 'good' gut bacteria can control genes in our cells. They demonstrated that chemical messages from the gut bacteria can alter chemical markers through the entire human genome. This interaction suggests that gut bacteria could potentially play an infection-fighting role.

Working alongside our genome, we have the epigenome, which is a set of chemical switches and markers that influence gene activity and expression. The epigenome is influenced by environmental factors, such as diet, physical activity, stress and sleep.

Referred to as 'epigenetic modifications', when these chemicals are placed on parts of the DNA or associated proteins, they influence their role and function. A direct consequence of these modifications is that genes can be switched on or off. Recent studies have shown that short-chain fatty acids (SCFAs), such as butyrate, which are produced when our gut microbes digest fibre-rich fruit and vegetables, can in fact influence these modifications.

In a study, researchers found that feeding mice with a diet that was rich in sugar and fat, but deficient in fibre, led to significant changes. The researchers observed that the mice had significantly reduced levels of Bacteroidetes and a greater amount of Firmicutes (two common

types of bacteria) compared to mice fed a fibre-rich diet. As we will learn shortly, this isn't a good thing, as having high levels of Firmicutes has been associated with a greater risk of obesity, while reduced levels of Bacteroidetes is associated with higher levels of inflammation in the gut. These findings emphasize the importance of diet on the composition of our gut bacteria.

Further recent studies have established a link between the gut microbiota, epigenetics and the occurrence of conditions such as immune disorders, inflammatory bowel diseases and even cancer.

A shout-out for butyrate

Butyrate is a very special SCFA. It has significant anti-inflammatory powers that promote the mucus we need in order to protect our gut lining. This is paramount, as without a healthy gut lining our immunity, skin and mental health can suffer. A damaged gut lining can also result in 'leaky gut'. Unlike most other cells in your body, which use glucose as their main energy source, the cells of the lining of your gut mainly use butyrate. Without it, these cells can't perform their functions adequately. It also keeps inflammation at bay, our gut cells healthy and our 'good' gut bacteria species, such as Bacteroidetes, thriving.

> **LEAKY GUT** is when toxins or particles of undigested food escape into the bloodstream, which can lead to impaired immunity, IBS, mood issues, skin problems and allergy-type symptoms.

Diversity is key

We need lots of variety when it comes to gut bacteria, so it is important to make sure our guts have as many different bacteria species as possible. This can be achieved by eating a variety of different foods, rich in different species of bacteria – all of which promote a healthy gut lining and balanced microbiome, in addition to healthy and balanced immunity.

Beneficial gut bacteria species have been demonstrated to impact both the innate and acquired immune systems. They have also been shown to shorten the duration of having a common cold, and decrease the severity of the symptoms. However, if you have ever had antibiotics, chances are a lot of your 'good' bacteria have been wiped out. Certain antibiotics can induce long-term changes to the gut microbiota. In fact, just one antibiotic treatment may lead to adverse changes in the composition and diversity of the microbiota. In comparison with our ancestors, who survived without antibiotics, we only have a tiny proportion of the diversity of gut bacteria species they had.

Our microbes educate and 'train' our immunity from the day we are born, and this may explain the 'hygiene hypothesis', which maintains that being too clean, especially in infancy, results in less exposure to different microbes and a subsequent reduction in microbiota diversity. This can also mean that the diversity in the development and education of the immune system is decreased as well, and may be one reason why autoimmune disease and allergies are increasing to critical levels.

When the microbiome malfunctions

Two of the main potential problems that may result when our gut health goes awry are 'dysbiosis' and impaired intestinal permeability, a.k.a. 'leaky gut'. These can lead to impaired immunity, painful gut symptoms and illness.

Dysbiosis

When our gut microbiota and microbiome is imbalanced this is known as 'dysbiosis'. This is mainly due to the increasing presence of harmful bacteria. It has also been reported that dysbiosis may be influencing how well messages are being sent via the gut-brain axis, by promoting inflammation and triggering our gut lining to become more permeable. This means more foods may be entering the intestine undigested, resulting in 'leaky gut' (see below), and painful consequences such as gas, diarrhoea, constipation and bloating. Not chewing our food properly may also result in undigested particles of food reaching the large intestine, where the harmful microbes may feed on it and then multiply. Furthermore, dysbiosis can also lead to systemic inflammation, which has been associated with autoimmune disease.

Leaky gut

Leaky gut occurs when the tight junctions of your intestinal wall loosen, which may then allow harmful bacteria, toxins or particles of undigested food to escape into the bloodstream. This can lead to impaired immunity, pain, fatigue, IBS, mood issues, skin problems and allergy-type symptoms. There are numerous reasons why leaky gut can occur, including after antibiotic treatment, a gut infection, or as a result of a nutrient-deficient diet. Our gut barrier is meant to keep 'invaders' out, but when the tight junctions loosen, the 'invaders' can enter and wreak havoc. This highlights the importance of ensuring we have sufficient amounts of our 'good' gut bacteria and also diversity, since these beneficial bacteria help to strengthen our gut barrier. Without a strong gut barrier, our immune system may begin to mount an immune response if these toxins and undigested particles of food enter the blood stream.

A healthy gut microbiome has been demonstrated to help prevent leaky gut syndrome and even reverse the condition if you do find yourself suffering from it. By embarking on the gut repair programme in the next chapter (see page 31), gut irritants will be removed, thus allowing your gut to begin to repair.

How healthy is your gut and immune system?

The following questionnaire, which looks at various symptoms and lifestyle factors, will give you a good idea as to how healthy your gut is and how balanced your immunity is at present.

Score 1 point for each time you answer 'yes'.

Part 1 – General health

1. Do you suffer from more than three or four colds a year?

2. Do you struggle to get rid of a cold, flu or infection?

3. Do you have a treatment or course of antibiotics two or more times a year?

4. Do you take regular medication?

5. Do you suffer from an allergy?

6. Do you suffer from hay fever?

7. Do you suffer from asthma?

8. Do you have arthritis?

9. Do you have eczema or psoriasis?

10. Do you regularly get cystitis or thrush?

11. Have you had cancer, or is there a family history of cancer?

Part 2 – Daily diet

1. Do you need caffeine to get you going in the morning?

2. Do you rely on a stimulant, such as caffeine/cigarettes/sugar, to get you through the day?

3. Do you drink more than 2 units of alcohol a day?

4. Do you consume less than 1.5 litres (50fl oz) of fluid a day?

5. Do you consume processed foods daily?

6. Do you eat less than three vegetable servings and two fruit servings a day?

7. Do you eat red meat more than three times per week?

8. Do you feel you need to snack in between meals?

9. Do you feel tired after eating during the day, especially after lunch?

10. Do you frequently eat when stressed?

11. Do you often eat 'on the go'?

Part 3 – Lifestyle

1. Are you overweight, with a BMI of over 25?

2. Do you exercise for less than 30 minutes five times a week (a 30-minute moderate walk, for example)?

3. Does your work involve sitting for long periods of time?

4. Are you exposed to natural sunlight for less than 10–15 minutes most days?

5. Do you smoke or are you regularly exposed to second-hand smoke?

6. Do you suffer from insomnia or other sleep issues?

7. Are you prone to getting angry?

8. Do you find yourself getting upset easily?

9. Do you suffer from anxiety?

10. Have you suffered a bereavement in the last 12 months, or a significant loss of any kind?

Once you have answered this questionnaire, please add up all your 'yes' answers and refer to the points system below.

20+

If you want to achieve a strong and healthy gut and immune system, you should make substantial modifications to your lifestyle and diet. This book will guide you on how to embrace and implement these changes, but in addition you may want to see a dietician or registered nutritionist who can help you further.

10+

Your gut and immune system is likely to be performing satisfactorily, but not at its optimum. Focus on working on the areas where you have answered 'yes' to support your gut and immune system. This book will guide you on how to embrace and implement these changes.

9 and below

Well done – it sounds as though you have good gut health and a healthy and efficient immune system. To support your gut health and immune system even further, check where you answered 'yes' and focus on making changes to these areas. This book will guide you on how to embrace and implement these changes.

Our gut microbiome plays a key role in our immunity, and the interaction between our gut microbiome and immune system is ultimately what maintains our health. Moreover, the foods we choose to consume influence not only our gut bacteria, but also our immunity. Strengthening our immune system is vital to fight infection, reduce our risk of autoimmune disease and allergies, as well as preventing chronic disease.

It is very clear that one of the most important factors for a healthy immune system is good gut health, and the next chapter will guide you on this journey. You will learn how to repair and transform the health of your gut, which in turn will help promote strong and balanced immunity.

part 2:
the most effective strategies

chapter 5:
diet – repair your gut first

The first key principle when it comes to restoring good gut health is to focus on repairing it. The following is a straightforward programme, which can help to improve gut health and involves several phases. However, before you embark on this gut health-restoring programme, it can be helpful to keep a food and symptoms journal for seven days, so you can spot any specific foods that may be the cause of your symptoms. Furthermore, if you have an existing medical condition, I advise speaking to a medical practitioner before embarking on this programme.

Phase one – remove

This first phase generally lasts 2–4 weeks, depending on your symptoms. We want to focus on repairing, and the initial step in this phase is to remove any foods and chemicals that you think may be causing you digestive discomfort. This includes foods that disturb the gut microbiota and cause intestinal permeability, a.k.a. leaky gut (see page 27). It also includes chemicals that harm the beneficial gut bacteria.

Foods that are a common cause of gut issues include dairy, eggs, gluten, soy, shellfish and coffee.

Therefore, in this phase, focus on removing the following foods from your diet:

- Dairy products

- Very fibrous vegetables, such as broccoli, Brussels sprouts and cabbage (these can cause bloating, but can be re-introduced after 2 weeks)

- Gluten and refined grains

- Alcohol

- Coffee (if it causes digestive issues)

- Legumes and pulses (e.g. beans, lentils and soybeans – they contain lectin, which can cause bloating)

As you will see, I have recommended the removal of legumes in this phase, since they can cause bloating. In addition, researchers have suggested that the lectins they contain can cause increased gut permeability, and possibly drive autoimmune diseases. However, you are able to re-introduce these after two weeks, and it is important to do so if you are vegan, as legumes are a great plant protein source.

> **LECTINS** are a family of carbohydrate-binding proteins, which occur in nearly all foods, but the highest amounts are found in legumes.

I don't recommend removing too many foods at once; instead, remove in stages, starting with the food that you suspect is the number-one culprit causing your symptoms.

I have suggested you may wish to remove coffee during this phase. Caffeine can be problematic for some people, as it is a stimulant and can promote the release of the stress hormones cortisol and adrenaline. However, research has shown that your genes have a major influence on your tolerance to it. Some people can consume significantly more than others without negative effects. If you feel jittery after consuming coffee, I would eliminating it during this phase.

This phase also involves removing chemicals, since they are harmful to the gut. These include dietary chemicals, such as artificial sweeteners, additives and preservatives, as well as the chemicals produced by our own bodies, such as excessive cortisol, a.k.a. the stress hormone. Chronic stress, which we will look at further in Chapter 10: how to manage stress effectively (see pages 53–55), has a significant and adverse impact on our gut health and immunity.

What can we eat in this initial phase?

• Vegetables (and some fruit) – focus on filling half your plate with vegetables, which provide with great sources of carbohydrate. Aim for lots of colour as variety is vital for optimum gut health and immunity. In addition, vegetables and fruit are packed with phytochemicals, also known as phytonutrients. These are powerful plant compounds that have antioxidant, anti-inflammatory and anti-microbial properties.

• Protein – focus on good-quality protein sources, which are vital for repairing the gut lining, e.g. fatty fish (wild salmon, mackerel, sardines), eggs, chicken, soy, tofu, tempeh, nuts.

• Healthy fats – concentrate on non-dairy fats, such as the monounsaturated fats found in olive oil, avocado, nuts and seeds. Additionally, coconut oil can be beneficial for your gut, as the medium-chain fatty acids (MCFAs) present in coconut oil are easier to digest than some other fats. This may be preferable if you have a leaky gut, or a gut that needs extra support. And while coconut oil is made up of about 90% saturated fat, it differs from the saturated fats found in animal fats, since more than 50% of the fats in coconut oil are healthy MCFAs, such as lauric acid. In fact, coconut oil is the highest natural source of lauric acid.

• Herbs and spices – these are rich in polyphenols, which are a category of plant compounds that provide numerous health benefits, including maintaining gut health. Furthermore, polyphenols have been shown to act on the gut microbiota by increasing the growth of beneficial bacteria, while inhibiting the growth of pathogens (harmful bacteria), thus exerting prebiotic-like effects.

How much protein do we need?

· In the UK, an average daily requirement of 0.6g protein per kilogram of body weight is estimated for adults. The adult Reference Nutrient Intake (RNI) is set at 0.75g of protein per kilogram of body weight per day. This equates to approximately 56g per day for men and 45g per day for women, aged 19–50 years respectively.

· Protein recommendations are similar in the US, where the DRI (Dietary Reference Intake) is 0.8 grams of protein per kilogram of body weight. This amounts to 56g per day for the average sedentary man, and 46g per day for the equivalent woman.

*However, protein requirements are increased for physically active individuals, as well as in older people, and those recovering from injuries.

During Phase 1, we need to focus on repairing the gut lining and ensuring adequate intake of nutrients, such as vitamins A and D, zinc, omega-3 fatty acids and antioxidants, which is also explored further in Chapter 7: eat to improve your immunity – the micros and phytonutrients (see pages 42–48). Ensure you get plenty of the following:

Vitamin A – found in sweet potatoes, butternut squash and pumpkin.

Vitamin D – found in wild salmon, sardines, herrings, egg yolks and mushrooms.

Zinc – found in shellfish, hemp seeds, pumpkin seeds, sesame seeds, nuts and eggs.

Antioxidants – found in red, purple, yellow, orange and green fruit and vegetables, and green and white tea.

Nutritional anti-inflammatories – such as omega-3 fatty acids (found in fatty fish, nuts and seeds) and curcumin (the main active ingredient in turmeric), which has powerful anti-inflammatory effects and is also a potent antioxidant.

Bone broth – an excellent restorative for the GI mucosa, it contains collagen and the amino acids glycine and glutamine, which are nutrients that can really help repair the gut lining.

You may feel better after two weeks on this phase, but you may wish to continue for up to four weeks.

Phase two – re-introduce

Once you have completed the initial 2–4-week phase, you can begin to re-introduce the foods you removed in Phase 1. Introduce each food one by one, over the course of three days. If symptoms reappear after you introduce a particular food, eliminate it, leave it a few days, then re-introduce a different food. Remember, you can re-introduce pulses at this point, which are rich in prebiotic fibre, but you must ensure you introduce them slowly.

When it comes to gluten, I suggest starting with sourdough bread, since the wild yeast and lactobacilli in the leaven neutralize the phytic acid, thereby making it a lot easier to digest. Then, introduce the 'lower' gluten grains, such as rye, and finally introduce wheat over three days.

With dairy, I would advise starting with live natural yoghurt, cheese, butter and then milk (in that order).

During this phase, you can re-introduce alcohol in moderation. I recommend opting for red wine, as it is loaded with antioxidants, and enjoying a glass with your dinner. The powerful plant compounds in red wine have been associated with numerous health benefits, including reduced inflammation, decreased risk of heart disease and cancer, and even longevity. Furthermore, red wine has been demonstrated to increase the abundance of beneficial gut bacteria, while reducing the number of harmful gut bacteria. This indicates the potentially beneficial prebiotic effects associated with red wine polyphenols.

Prebiotics and probiotics

At this stage, I recommend you increase your intake of pre- and probiotic foods.

Prebiotics
A prebiotic is a type of dietary fibre that feeds your 'good' gut bacteria. Many people think prebiotics and fibre are the same thing, but they're not! To be classed as a prebiotic, the fibre must:

- Not be absorbed in the gastrointestinal tract;

- Be able to be fermented by gut bacteria;

- Promote the growth and activity of certain beneficial bacteria to improve health[46].

In addition, prebiotic fibre helps our bacteria make certain nutrients, such as butyrate (see page 26), for the cells in the large intestine. This then promotes a healthier and balanced gastrointestinal tract.

As you will see in Part 3, lots of the prebiotic-rich foods that I highlight in the table over the page feature frequently in the recipes.

Seeds such as flax (linseeds), hemp seeds and chia seeds, which have been sprouted, are also excellent sources of fibre and help 'feed' the good bacteria. However, if you have a weakened and damaged gut, you may wish to get your fibre from steamed vegetables and fruit initially. Then, you can introduce sprouted seeds when your gut is feeling stronger.

Vegetables	Fruit	Nuts, seeds and legumes	Miscellaneous
Asparagus Jerusalem artichokes Beetroot (beets) Chicory (endive) Cauliflower Cold potatoes Leeks Onions Pak choi (bok choy)	Apples Apricots Bananas Grapefruit Nectarines Persimmon Tomatoes Watermelon White peaches	Almonds Cashew nuts Chia seeds Flax seeds (linseeds) Pistachios Black beans Butter (lima) beans Chickpeas (garbanzo beans) Lentils	Apple cider vinegar Barley Cocoa (70% dark chocolate) Fresh root ginger Oats Quinoa Raw honey Rye Wild rice

Probiotics

These are the live bacteria found in certain foods or supplements that can provide numerous health benefits, including promoting digestive health and supporting our immunity. During this phase and going forward, focus on including fermented foods, which contain probiotic bacteria, such as live yoghurt, sauerkraut, kimchi and kefir.

I get asked a lot if it is worth supplementing with probiotics. The main issue when it to comes to probiotics is that research is still in its infancy, and we don't know as yet which exact strains should be taken and if they are helpful for all individuals. If you are very young, old or very ill, there is a growing body of research that suggests they are beneficial[47]. However, if this doesn't apply to you, I would recommend concentrating on promoting your beneficial gut bacteria by consuming a diverse, fibre-rich diet.

Glutamine

This is the most abundant amino acid (building block of protein) in the body, and it plays a vital role in gut health. It encourages immune-cell activity in the gut, helps prevent infection and inflammation, and heals the gut lining. The best food sources of glutamine include beetroot (beets), cabbage, spinach, tofu, lentils, beans, bone broth, chicken and fish.

Digestive Aids

You may find that you need to replace naturally occurring digestive aids, including enzymes, hydrochloric acid and bile acids that support proper digestion. These can be taken in supplement form before eating a meal, but I would suggest seeking advice from a nutritionist or dietician if you suspect you may need them. They can advise you further and ensure you are taking the appropriate digestive aid.

chapter 6:
eat to improve your immunity – the macros

Macronutrients are nutrients that we need daily in fairly large quantities. They include proteins, carbohydrates and lipids (fat). They provide our bodies with energy, promote growth and repair, and support our immunity and numerous other areas of health. We need to make sure the macros in our diet are balanced, or it can have a significant and adverse effect on our immunity. The macros all have their own functions, although our immune cells alternate between carbs and fats as their fuel source. When we are fighting an infection, their choice of fuel is carbs, but for day-to-day functioning (when we are not battling a cold, fever or infection) our immune cells use fat.

A balanced and nutrient-dense diet is crucial to supporting our immune function. Research has shown that the development and optimal functioning of our immunity is directly influenced by diet. In addition, any deficiency or excess of certain nutrients can affect the number and activity of immune cells, thus balance is vital. As well as ensuring healthy immunity, a balanced diet is also key for promoting optimal gut health. Studies have shown that there is a significant amount of interaction between our body's immune system and the gut microbiota, and diet is considered to play a significant role in influencing our microbiota[48].

Lipids (a.k.a. fats)

Dietary fatty acids are said to have major effects on immunity, and studies have also demonstrated that nuts and other plant-based foods, which are abundant in polyunsaturated and mono-unsaturated fats, can increase gut bacteria diversity.

The groups of fatty acids that together form fat are called lipids, and are what I am referring to when I use the word 'fat' in relation to diet. Fat is as essential to your diet as protein and carbohydrates and has several important functions, such as being an essential building block for our cells, providing energy and the fat-soluble vitamins A, D, E and K. Fats are mainly produced in the liver, and come in a variety of forms to replenish the cells and provide energy for organs such as our brain.

However, not all fats are created equal:

- While some fats are associated with beneficial effects on health, others have been shown to be harmful.

- Diets high in fat have also been shown to alter gut bacteria and are associated with a decrease in the diversity of gut bacteria, which is not a good thing!

- Consuming too much fat of any kind can result in an abundance of excess calories, and an increase in body weight and body fat.

There are two types of fats that have been identified as potentially harmful to your health: saturated fat and trans fats.

Saturated fat

Saturated fats tend to be solid at room temperature and are found in fatty cuts of beef, pork, poultry skin, lard and high-fat dairy foods, such as full-fat (whole) milk, butter and cheese.

In a paper published in the journal, *Cell Reports*[49], researchers found that saturated fat can 'short-circuit' both mouse and human immune cells, producing an inappropriate inflammatory response as a consequence. Furthermore, a review of 15 randomized controlled trials (RCT – the gold standard when it comes to evidence) that investigated saturated fats and heart disease concluded that replacing saturated fat in your diet with healthier polyunsaturated fats may reduce heart disease risk[50].

According to the British Nutrition Foundation[51], even though significant progress has been achieved in working towards the target of getting population intakes of saturated fat below 11 per cent of food energy, there is still quite a way to go. However, there are several easy ways to cut down on the amount of saturated fat in the diet, including:

• Choosing lower-fat meats such as turkey and chicken;

• Removing all skin and fat from meat;

• Opting for 'healthy' fats, such as olive oil, which are richer in monounsaturated fatty acids.

Monounsaturated fat

Monounsaturated fats, also referred to as MUFAs, are seen as one of the 'good' fats able to decrease inflammation and support our immunity. They come mainly from olive oil and rapeseed (canola) oil, but are also found in plant foods like avocados and nuts, as well as meat and animal products. The American Heart Association recommends that the majority of fats you eat should be monounsaturated or polyunsaturated, instead of saturated and trans fats[52].

Polyunsaturated fat

Polyunsaturated fats, also referred to as PUFAs, are essential fatty acids, which means they're essential for normal body functions. As your body can't make them, you must get them from food. PUFAs help with blood clotting and are also involved in the composition of cell membranes. In addition, they play a very important role in regulating the nervous system, blood pressure and inflammation. The most common types of PUFA oils are sunflower oil and safflower oil.

In their unheated form, PUFAs have been reported to reduce the risk of heart disease, support immunity and exert various other health benefits. However, when they are heated these beneficial effects are cancelled out. Damaged polyunsaturated fats are called 'trans fats' and they are the worst type of dietary fat, shown to impact immunity and also fertility in women. There is no safe level of trans fats; therefore they have been officially banned in the United States, Denmark, Austria and Switzerland. Currently, trans fats aren't banned in the UK; however, the government has chosen to allow food companies to voluntarily reduce the trans-fat content in their products. Although many UK food producers have agreed to omit trans fats, it is believed that some foods still have them, often listed as 'mono and diglycerides of fatty acids', so do read food labels carefully.

Foods that may contain trans fats are typically sweet, carbohydrate-based foods or those with relatively short shelf lives.

Trans fats are typically present in the following foods:

· Margarines which contain hydrogenated vegetable oils

· Baked goods, such as bread, cakes, pastries and doughnuts

· Fast food

· Ice cream

There are two main types of PUFA: omega-3 and omega-6 fatty acids. These are both very important nutrients.

Omega-3 fatty acids

Omega-3 fats are known as essential fatty acids and must be derived from our diet as our bodies are unable to make them. They are required for essential functions such as digestion, cholesterol transportation, brain function and blood clotting. They are also vital for our immunity, as they may enhance the functioning of the immune cells.

Omega-3 fatty acids have been shown to decrease inflammation, and a significant body of research has consistently reported a link between a greater omega-3 intake and reduced inflammation. Inflammation is a natural response to infections and is crucial for our health, but when inflammation lasts for a long time it is referred to as 'chronic inflammation' and needs to be addressed. Studies have also shown that consuming a sufficient intake of omega-3s during the first year of life is associated with a decreased risk of autoimmunity. Additionally, these super-powerful nutrients have been observed to help treat lupus, rheumatoid arthritis, ulcerative colitis, Crohn's disease and psoriasis.

> **Chronic inflammation** has been shown to be a factor in nearly all chronic diseases in the Western world.

The three most important omega-3 fatty acids are: ALA, EPA and DHA. You can find ALA in plant-based foods such as walnuts, flax seeds (linseeds) and chia seeds, while you are most likely to find EPA and DHA in animal produce, such as wild salmon, mackerel and trout. We need to convert ALA into EPA or DHA for us to be able to actually use it for optimum health. However, in humans this process is inadequate, with approximately 1–10 per cent of ALA being successfully converted into EPA and 0.5–5 per cent being converted into DHA[53]. If it isn't converted, it can be used as an energy source or will be stored as fat.

Omega-6 fatty acids

Like omega-3 fatty acids, these are also essential and you need to get them from your diet. They can be found in most vegetable oils, nuts, fatty meat and some farmed fish fed on soy and corn. The most common omega-6 fat is linoleic acid, which can be converted into other omega-6 fats, including arachidonic acid. As with EPA, our important omega-3 friend, arachidonic acid generates eicosanoids; however, these are more pro-inflammatory, and if there are too many, it may result in increased inflammation.

Although omega-6 fats are essential in the right quantities, the optimal ratio of omega 3:6 has not been well defined, and there are differing views about the ideal ratio. However, recent research has suggested that to improve this ratio, we should focus on consuming more omega-3s in our diet, not less omega-6s. In the UK, intakes of omega-6 (principally linoleic acid) are close to the recommendation of 6.5 per cent of dietary energy[51]. However, the American Heart Association recommends getting 5–10 per cent of your daily calories from omega-6 fats[52].

Getting your omega-6 fats

What does 5–10 per cent of daily calories from omega-6 fats look like? Based on an individual who consumes 2,000 calories a day, this would equate to approximately 11–22g:

- Small handful of walnuts (about 30g/1oz) = 11g

- Salad dressing, made with 1 tablespoon safflower oil = 9g

- Small handful of flax seeds (linseeds) or sunflower seeds (these taste great sprinkled over a salad or yoghurt) = 9g

Getting your omega-3 fats

While there are currently no government guidelines in the UK as to how much omega-3 fat we should be eating, it is widely accepted that two portions of fatty fish per week is recommended. If you don't eat fish or are vegan, opt for algae supplements instead. Alternatively, you may wish to supplement, and this is covered in the next chapter (page 42).

Three of my favourite omega-3-rich recipes:

- Wild Salmon Veggie Bowl (page 122)

- Tangy Tuna Steaks (page 159)

- Anchovy and Tomato Risotto (page 151)

Carbs

Carbs have been vilified in recent years, yet we need carbs in our diet, as glucose is the major source of fuel for the brain and the immune system. We need to focus on prioritizing complex carbs that are rich in fibre, while limiting the highly refined simple sugars, which are found in sweets, chocolate and cakes. Simple carbs are energy-dense (high in calories), yet deficient in nutrients and quickly absorbed. Research has also shown that high-carbohydrate meals may lead to greater oxidative stress and inflammatory response[54].

Complex carbs

These healthful dietary components are made up of sugar molecules that are strung together in long, complex chains. While simple sugars, such as sucrose, are absorbed rapidly, complex carbs such as vegetables, legumes and whole grains tend to take longer to be metabolized, thus preventing blood-sugar spikes. They are also lower in calories, while being nutrient dense and providing us with vital vitamins, minerals, phytonutrients and fibre.

An animal model study[55] demonstrated that a high-fat, high-sugar diet has an adverse impact on our gut microbiome, which may influence the brain and behaviour. In addition, human studies have reported that artificial sweeteners can exert a negative effect on our blood glucose, because of their influence on our gut microbes. Furthermore, it was demonstrated that aspartame promotes the number of some bacterial strains that are associated with metabolic disease.

Metabolic disease refers to a group of conditions that can raise your risk of heart disease and Type-2 diabetes.

When we are fighting an infection, our immune cells' preferred source of fuel is glucose. If we don't have enough glucose, this can impact our immune system's ability to deal with an infection, and may lead to a reduction in number and function of crucial immune cells[56]. While balanced blood sugar is crucial for reducing chronic disease risk, it is also paramount for immunity. If blood sugar levels stay high for too long, this hinders our immune cells' ability to carry out their role and function, which makes us vulnerable to infections. To promote healthy blood-sugar balance, we need to focus on including the best-quality carbs possible, which as we know are the complex carbs (whole grains, beans and fruit). Complex carbs take longer to digest, which means they have less of an immediate impact on blood sugar, causing it to rise more slowly. In addition, they are highly nutritious and loaded with micronutrients, phytonutrients and fibre.

Fabulous fibre

In the 1970s and '80s, we discovered that there were two main types of fibre – insoluble and soluble. Unlike soluble fibre, insoluble fibre is not fermented in the colon and doesn't 'feed' our good bacteria. However, it is important to our health, and aids with more regular bowel movement. Soluble fibre 'feeds' our bacteria and helps them thrive, and this type of fibre has also been shown to switch immune cells from pro-inflammatory to anti-inflammatory, which helps us to heal faster from infection[57].

Prebiotic fibre is important for feeding our 'good' gut bacteria. If we don't eat enough prebiotic fibre, this results in an adverse effect on our immunity and may lead to illness[58]. Therefore, by feeding our gut bacteria, we are also strengthening our immune system.

Inulin and beta-glucan

Two other types of soluble fibre include inulin and beta-glucan, and these also promote the growth of our 'good' gut bacteria. Beta-glucan fibre can be found in oats and barley, and studies have shown that it can enhance immune response, as well has exerting anti-inflammatory and antimicrobial benefits[59]. Inulin-rich foods include onions, leeks, garlic, chicory (endive) and Jerusalem artichokes. In fact, over 70 per cent of the fibre in a Jerusalem artichoke comes from inulin. Unfortunately, people who are intolerant to FODMAP foods are likely to experience side effects from consuming these foods, such as gas and bloating. Therefore, when adding inulin-rich foods to your diet, start with small amounts, as larger amounts are more likely to trigger side effects. If you increase intake slowly over time, that will help the body to adjust.

FODMAP stands for 'fermentable oligosaccharides, disaccharides, mono-saccharides, and polyols'. They include sugars that may cause digestive discomfort in some people. FODMAP foods include wheat, garlic, onion, watermelon, apples, apricots, cherries, nectarines and plums.

Resistant starch

Another type of fibre is resistant starch, which provides the benefits of both insoluble and soluble fibre. It is also beneficial to our immunity and gut health to include resistant starch in our diets, which our gut bacteria love. This starch can't be digested anywhere except the colon – hence 'resistant'. Once it reaches the colon, it feeds the friendly gut bacteria, which then gobble it up and release butyrate. As we know, butyrate strengthens our gut lining, in addition to lowering inflammation. Foods such as cold white potatoes (they need to be cooked then cooled), unripe bananas, legumes and rice (cooked and cooled) are all good sources of resistant starch.

A healthy digestive tract is paramount for the immune system as, if we are continually constipated, there can be a build-up of toxins, which may then be absorbed into the bloodstream. The immune system then has to contend with this, as does the beneficial gut bacteria who move aside for types like Candida, which we want to limit. Without an adequate intake of fibre our immune system can't function properly. So, try to include as many different coloured vegetables on your plate as possible. Ideally, aim for 25–30 different vegetables (and some fruit) a week: research shows that those who consume a greater variety of plant-based foods have more diverse and healthier microbiomes. We don't yet know which gut bacteria prefer which foods, so include as much variety as possible.

- In the UK, a staggering 90 per cent of people do not eat enough fibre.

- The average intake is 17g per day for women and 20g per day for men[51].

- The actual recommended average intake for adults is 30g per day.

What does 30g of fibre look like?
Here's an example of how you can reach your 30g a day goal:

- 50g/2oz/½ cup rolled oats (oatmeal) = 9g

- 1 thick slice of wholegrain bread = 2g

- 1 apple = 4g

- 100g/3½oz/½ cup cooked lentils = 8g

- 25g/1oz/scant ¼ cup pistachio nuts = 3g

- 1 carrot = 3g

- 1 banana = 3g

I have included lots of recipes in the book that are rich in fibre, prebiotic fibre and resistant starch. Three of my favourite fibre-rich recipes:

- Overnight Chocolate Oats (page 71)

- Chickpea and Cumin Burgers (page 113)

- Veggie Cottage Pie with Sweet Potato Mash (page 135)

Key points

- Do increase fibre intake slowly to give your gut time to adapt.

- Include a variety of foods in your diet to ensure you are eating foods that contain the three main types of fibre – soluble, insoluble and resistant starch.

- Drink enough water, as this will help prevent constipation when increasing your fibre intake.

- Focus on foods in their natural state and ideally consume organic produce, if possible, as this has a significantly more diverse bacteria population than conventionally grown produce.

Protein

Proteins are large molecules that have numerous roles in our body. They are needed for the structure, function, growth and repair of our tissues and organs. Since all our cells contain protein, this powerful macronutrient is critical and helps to promote optimal health and strong immunity. It has been well-documented that protein deficiency damages immune function and increases the susceptibility of animals and humans to infectious disease[60].

The amino acids

Proteins are made up of lots of smaller molecules known as amino acids. These are all linked to each other in long chains. It is the order of amino acids that determines each protein's individual structure and its precise role and function.

There are 20 different types of amino acids that can be combined to make a protein, and our body makes 11 of these, referred to as 'non-essential amino acids'. However, there are nine known as 'essential amino acids' that you must consume in your daily diet because your body is unable to make them. In addition, our clever, friendly gut bacteria can make very small amounts for us.

Getting the right balance of amino acids is vital for our immunity since they are essential to making immune cells, cytokines and antibodies to fight infection.

Complete proteins
These provide all of the nine essential amino acids that your body needs in appropriate amounts. Meat, poultry, seafood, eggs and milk products are examples of complete proteins. When it comes to plant-based protein, I use

soy and quinoa a lot in my recipes, as they are considered a complete protein.

Incomplete proteins

These provide some amino acids, but not all of them. Many plant-based proteins are incomplete proteins, and must be consumed together as complementary proteins in order to get all of the amino acids that the body needs. Nuts, seeds and most grains are examples of incomplete proteins. However, by eating rice along with beans, lentils or tofu, you improve the balance of amino acids and increase the usability of the protein.

How much protein do we need?

Since too little protein in the diet may lead to symptoms of weakness, fatigue and poor immunity, it is vital we consume sufficient amounts. In the UK, men and women aged 19–50 need approximately 56g and 45g per day of protein, respectively. People over 65 may benefit from consuming a little more protein – between 1g and 1.2g per 1kg of their body weight – to help minimize age-related muscle loss[61].

Protein recommendations are similar in the US, where the recommended intake is 0.8g of protein per kilogram of body weight. This amounts to 56g per day for the average sedentary man, and 46g for the average sedentary woman. However, there are notable exceptions: anyone with severe kidney disease should avoid extra protein; also, weight-lifters and endurance athletes may need more to repair and rebuild their muscles.

What does 50g of protein in a day look like?

- 2 large eggs = 12g

- 100g/3½oz wild salmon fillet = 21g

- 1 serving of miso soup = 7g

- 50g/2oz/⅓ cup uncooked quinoa = 7g

- 100g/3½oz/scant ½ cup natural (plain) yoghurt = 4g

---

key points – nutrition to strengthen your immunity

1. Eat plenty of fibre-rich complex carbohydrates, such as oats, quinoa and brown rice. Fibre is a fantastic way to support immunity through your gut microbiome, while limiting refined sugar, as a high-sugar diet is harmful to our microbiomes. Bacteria love sugar, but if we consume a lot of sugar, the bacteria we don't want more of in our guts are likely to multiply and potentially lead to dysbiosis.

2. Aim for at least 7 servings of vegetables and fruit a day (at least 5 vegetables and 2 fruit servings). Try to get 25–30 or more different veggies a week on your plate.

3. Protein is important for immunity, so include diverse protein sources in your diet and include plant-based proteins, such as lentils, quinoa, beans or tofu. (Do make sure you combine plant-protein sources, such as beans with rice, or lentils with rice, to ensure optimal protein quality).

4. Opt for fatty fish, such as wild salmon, sardines, trout or mackerel twice a week, or alternatively take an algae supplement if you don't eat fish (choosing fish over red meat helps to reduce our saturated fat intake). Fish is also the number-one source of omega-3 fatty acids, particularly in the case of fatty fish.

5. Include at least 1 tablespoon of seeds or cold-pressed oil a day (olive oil or avocado oil over salads work well).

6. Add spices and herbs to dishes – as well as bringing delicious flavour, spices and herbs have antioxidant and anti-inflammatory properties.

7. Try to eat organically where possible, and always consume foods in their natural state.

chapter 7:
eat to improve your immunity – the micros and phytonutrients

The wide range of nutrients involved in supporting immunity indicates that a nutritious, balanced and diverse diet is key. There are 13 vitamins and 20 minerals, and we need to meet all these micronutrient requirements to ensure our immune system is able to perform at its best. Various micronutrient deficiencies can have a significant and negative impact on our immunity, thereby increasing our risk of infection and disease. Let's have a look at the key vitamins and minerals involved in strengthening our immunity.

The vitamins

Vitamin A

This micronutrient plays an important role in our immunity, as it helps maintain an active thymus, which is key for strong immunity. Also, vitamin A is a potent antiviral vitamin as it helps to make cell walls stronger and more resistant to viral infection. Furthermore, the immune-system cells need vitamin A for lysozyme production, which is an antibacterial enzyme. Vitamin A is known as an anti-inflammatory vitamin because of its critical role in enhancing immune function[62]. It plays a vital role in helping to keep the skin, the lining of the respiratory system and the gut healthy, thereby protecting us from infections. Along with vitamin D and zinc, vitamin A is crucial for the health of the gut barrier. It also helps to maintain vision, particularly in dim light, and support growth. When you are fighting an infection, you need more vitamin A, and you may also require more if you are a smoker, experiencing intense stress, or are exposed to pollution.

Vitamin A derived from animal sources is called retinol, and that from plant-based sources is carotenoids. Retinol is more bioavailable, since the body has to convert carotenoids to retinol.

How much do we need a day?

In the UK, government guidelines for adults aged 19–64 is 0.7mg per day for men and 0.6mg per day for women. You should be able to get all the vitamin A you need from your diet. Also, any vitamin A your body doesn't need immediately is stored for future use, which means you don't need it every day.

In the US, recommendations are slightly different. The National Institutes of Health advise that the recommended daily amount (RDA) is actually given as retinol activity equivalents (RAE) to allow for the different bioactivities of retinol and provitamin A carotenoids – all are converted into retinol by the body[63]. For adults aged 19 and over, the guidelines are 900mcg (RAE) and 700mcg (RAE) per day for men and women, respectively.

Which foods can vitamin A be found in?
Rich food sources of vitamin A include beef liver, carrots, sweet potatoes, squash, mango, watercress, cantaloupe melon and pumpkin.

Should you supplement?
Studies have shown that consuming in excess of approximately 1.5mg a day of vitamin A over a long time may adversely impact bone health, putting you at an increased risk of fracture as you get older. Therefore, if you do take a multivitamin containing vitamin A, just check that your intake from supplements and food together doesn't exceed 1.5mg per day. If you eat liver or liver pâté more than once a week, be cautious, as you may be getting too much vitamin A.

Vitamin C

Vitamin C, also known as ascorbic acid, has an essential and extensive role in the immune system. Numerous studies have reported that vitamin C has powerful antimicrobial properties, which decrease infection risk, as well as exerting immunomodulatory functions[64]. Research has shown that a deficiency of the vitamin appears to make you more susceptible to infection. Some research suggests that, although regular vitamin-C intake likely won't prevent you from catching a cold, it may decrease the duration or severity of cold symptoms. A review of 31 studies found that consuming 1–2g of vitamin C daily reduced cold duration by 18 per cent in children and 8 per cent in adults. The review also confirmed that vitamin C may be beneficial for individuals who undergo brief periods of intense physical exercise[65].

As well as supporting our immune system, vitamin C has an important role in helping to protect the cells in our body. This potent antioxidant helps to heal wounds and maintain skin health, as well as helping to keep our blood vessels, bones and cartilage in tip-top condition. In addition, it's known that vitamin C increases iron absorption; thus, individuals with iron deficiency might benefit from increasing their vitamin C intake.

How much do we need a day?
In the UK, government guidelines for adults aged 19–64 is 40mg a day. You should be able to get all the vitamin C you need from your daily diet. Unlike vitamin A, it can't be stored in the body, so you need it in your diet every day. As we get older, our absorption of vitamin C decreases significantly, so older people need to increase their vitamin C intake, and spread it out over the course of the day.

In the US, the RDA for men aged 19 and over is 90mg a day, and for adult women it is 75mg a day. Pregnant women are advised to have 85mg of vitamin C a day, while 120mg a day is recommended during breastfeeding. Furthermore, US guidelines suggest that smokers need 35mg of vitamin C more a day, compared with those who don't smoke.

What foods can vitamin C be found in?
Foods rich in vitamin C include kiwi fruit, guavas, yellow and red (bell) peppers, blackcurrants, red chillies, broccoli, tomatoes, cabbage, cauliflower, strawberries and oranges.

Should you supplement?
Whether to supplement completely depends on your individual circumstances. Supplementing with 1–3g a day has been reported to have benefits if you are battling a cold, such as decreasing the severity of symptoms and reducing recovery times.

Vitamin D

This micronutrient is super-important for maintaining a strong immune system, with research indicating that vitamin D is involved in the activation of our important T cells, by 'priming' them ready to fight infection[66]. Furthermore, vitamin D has been shown to regulate gene expression and have an immunomodulatory influence on our immune cells. This powerful micronutrient can also promote the function of our NKT cells, increase Treg activity and inhibit Th1[67].

The body creates vitamin D from sunlight on the skin, and from springtime to mid autumn the majority of us should be able to get the vitamin D we need from sunlight. However, mid autumn and spring, we may not be able to get enough vitamin D from sunlight alone, even if we regularly spend time outside, which could result in deficiency.

Vitamin D deficiency can lead to rickets in children, which is a bone deformity, and a condition called osteomalacia in adults. Taking a vitamin D supplement in winter may be recommended for some individuals, especially if a blood check highlights you may be low in this essential micronutrient.

bones, teeth and muscles stay healthy. We will explore the role of vitamin D in more detail in Chapter 12 (page 59).

How much do we need a day?

In its report 'Vitamin D and Health', the Scientific Advisory Committee on Nutrition (SACN) recommends that Recommended Nutrient Intake (RNI) for all people ages 4 and over is 10mcg per day. For younger children and infants, the SACN advised that (as data are insufficient to set an RNI) a 'safe intake' of 8.5–10mcg per day has been set.

In the US, the RDA for adults aged 19–70 years is 600 IU (15mcg) for both men and women.

Groups at risk of low vitamin D include:

- Pregnant and breastfeeding women

- Older people over the age of 65

- Children and adolescents who spend little time outside

- People with darker skin tones – individuals of Asian, African, Afro-Caribbean and Middle Eastern descent – living in northern climates

- Those who cover their skin when outside or spend little time outside during the summer

---

25-hydroxyvitamin D (25(OH)D) is commonly considered as the best indicator of vitamin D status in the body.

In addition, vitamin D deficiency has long been associated with systemic autoimmune disease and is prevalent in multiple autoimmune diseases such as multiple sclerosis, Type-1 diabetes and lupus. Vitamin D status is associated with the risk of autoimmunity, therefore this potent micronutrient could be useful in potentially preventing and protecting you from autoimmune diseases.

As well as supporting our immunity, vitamin D has several other important functions, such as regulating the amount of calcium and phosphate in the body. These nutrients are required to help

Storage of vitamin D and 25(OH)D in adipose and other tissues has been well documented[68]. This could, in part, explain why serum 25(OH)D levels do not fall to critically low levels during the winter. So, in theory, you could stock up on it during the summer and early autumn ready for the start of the cold and flu season.

Which foods can vitamin D be found in?

Foods that contain good amounts of vitamin D include oily fish, e.g. wild salmon, herring, mackerel, sardines. Egg yolk and meat contain small amounts; some breakfast cereals contain added vitamin D. Increase vitamin D levels further by exposing mushrooms to ultraviolet light.

Should you supplement?

In the UK and parts of the US, it can be tricky to get our daily requirements of vitamin D all year round, since the sun isn't strong enough in the winter to allow us to make it. If you do opt to supplement, then 10mcg each day should be enough. If you are pregnant, be aware that while cod liver oil can be a good source of vitamin D, it also contains a lot of vitamin A, so do avoid cod liver oil if you are pregnant.

Vitamin E

Vitamin E is a fat-soluble vitamin that protects our cell membranes from damage, and the α-tocopherol form of this micronutrient particularly protects against cellular damage. We want to limit cellular damage as much as possible as it may lead to 'improper' immune response. Vitamin E is a powerful antioxidant that protects us from oxidative stress, and also has the ability to modulate immune functions.

How much do we need a day?
The UK government guidelines for adults aged 19–64 is 4mg per day for men and 3mg per day for women. You should be able to get all the vitamin E you need from your diet. Also, any vitamin E your body doesn't need immediately is stored for future use, which means you don't need it every day.

In the US, the RDA for individuals aged 14 and over is 15mg a day.

Which foods can vitamin E be found in?
Good sources of vitamin E include nuts and seeds, olive oil, wheat germ oil and avocado.

Should you supplement?
Most people who live in the UK and other developed nations, meet their vitamin E requirements through their diet. However, some digestive conditions, such as Crohn's disease and coeliac disease can hinder fat absorption, and individuals who suffer from these diseases may experience vitamin E deficiency. The US National Institutes of Health (NIH) state that supplementing with high doses of vitamin E can lead to adverse side effects, including one very serious side effect – haemorrhagic stroke[69].

Therefore, if you do suffer from a digestive condition, it would be advisable to speak with a dietician or nutritionist who can advise whether you may need to supplement.

Zinc

Zinc is a mineral and powerful antioxidant that is vital for strong immunity. It is a key player in cellular metabolism, and is needed for enzyme activity, protein and DNA synthesis as well as cell division. Zinc also supports wound healing, and growth and development during childhood. It is also very important in pregnancy, as it helps to build baby's cells and DNA. Zinc is critical for immune function, and for the development and function of cells that mediate our immunity[70]. Zinc deficiency has been shown to compromise the number and function of lymphocytes, with T cells being particularly vulnerable to zinc deficiency[71]. A deficiency in zinc causes the thymus to shrink, leading to low numbers of T cells, and can alter cytokine production, leading to oxidative stress and inflammation.

Even mild zinc deficiency, which is more common than severe zinc deficiency, can suppress aspects of immunity[72]. The elderly may be particularly at risk of deficiency given that there is a high prevalence of inadequate dietary zinc intake among those 60 years of age and older, and that plasma zinc concentration declines with age. It is not known why plasma zinc declines, but weakened absorption and epigenetic dysregulation may be contributing factors. Several RCTs (the gold standard in clinical trials) suggest that supplementation with low to moderate doses of zinc (10–45mg zinc/day) in healthy elderly individuals improves immune function.

How much do we need a day?
In the UK, government guidelines for men and women aged 19–64 is 9.5mg and 7mg per day, respectively.

In the US, 11mg for men and 8mg for women are the recommended daily intakes.

You should be able to get all the zinc you need from your daily diet. However, as zinc is not stored in the body, regular dietary intake is important to maintain normal functioning.

What foods can zinc be found in?
Oysters contain more zinc per serving than any other food, but red meat, poultry and shellfish provide the majority of zinc in the average Western diet. Other good food sources include beans, nuts, wholegrains, pumpkin seeds and dairy products. Phytates that are present in wholegrain breads, cereals, legumes and other foods can inhibit its absorption. Thus, the bioavailability of zinc from grains and plant foods is lower than that from animal foods, although many grain and plant-based foods are still good sources of zinc.

Should you supplement?
The Department of Health (UK) recommends that zinc intake should not be over 25mg per day. Furthermore, high doses of zinc reduce the amount of copper the body can absorb, which can lead to anaemia and weakening of the bones. So, just make sure you are staying within the guidelines.

Selenium

Selenium is another mineral and antioxidant that is critical for immune function, and is involved in the production of antibodies. In addition, selenium helps to regulate the production of cytokines and eicosanoids, which are involved in immune response.

Selenium deficiency has been shown to impair aspects of both the innate and adaptive immunity, and has been reported to promote the severity or progression of some viral infections[73].

> **An antioxidant** is a molecule that prevents or lessens the damage caused by free radicals and other oxidants.

How much do we need a day?
In the UK, government guidelines for men and women aged 19–64 is 75mcg and 60mcg per day, respectively. If you eat meat, fish or nuts, you should be able to get all the selenium you need from your daily diet.

In the US, the RDA for individuals over the age of 14 is 55mcg, while 60mcg is recommended during pregnancy, and 70mcg for breastfeeding mothers.

What foods can selenium be found in?
Rich sources of selenium include: Brazil nuts, sesame seeds, wholegrains and seafood.

Should you supplement?
Selenium influences immune response in various ways, and whether to supplement entirely depends on your individual circumstances. Supplementation has been reported to enhance cell-mediated immunity in those who may be deficient, and also strengthen the response to viruses. In contrast, supplementation has been shown to exacerbate allergic asthma and weaken the immune response to parasites[74]. Nutrition and supplementation is completely personalized, so you may wish to speak with a nutritionist or dietician.

The deal with supplementation

Should I supplement or not? I get asked this question almost every single day!

The first step towards improving your vitamin and mineral status is to focus on including a good variety of the foods mentioned, which are rich in the essential vitamins and minerals that are crucial to our immunity and health. Whether to supplement depends on your individual circumstances – nutrition has to be personalized.

The one supplement I do recommend for people over 60 is vitamin B12, since this micronutrient becomes harder to absorb as we age. I also recommend B12 for those who follow a vegan diet. Additionally, if you are elderly, or under a lot of physical or emotional stress, you may wish to take an all-round, high-quality multivitamin supplement. In a randomized control trial, elderly individuals who took a multivitamin experienced half the number of infections. They also gained considerable improvements in the strength and integrity of their immunity[75]. Therefore, supplementation may help elderly individuals maintain stronger immunity.

However, for most people, I would advise focusing on getting your nutrients from your diet first. We know that an excess of certain micronutrients can result in harmful side effects, and several studies have confirmed that taking high-dose supplements of vitamins A, C, D, E and folic acid is not always helpful for disease prevention, and it can even be damaging to health[76]. Furthermore, the long term health consequences of vitamin and mineral consumption are still unknown.

Vitamins and minerals for strong immunity

These micronutrient recommendations are based on the daily UK government guidelines for an average adult aged 19–64.

Phytochemicals

Phytochemicals, also known as phytonutrients, are compounds produced by plants, which have been shown to be beneficial for our health. Studies have reported they can reduce inflammation and fight harmful free radicals, thus helping to nourish our immunity and maintain good gut health.

There are many phytochemicals providing lots of different health benefits:

Polyphenols such as carotenoids support immune function, eye health and have also been shown to decrease cancer risk. There are hundreds of different carotenoids, including beta-carotene, lutein and lycopene. It is best to eat a carotenoid-food with a fat source, since this will promote optimal absorption. Carotenoids can be found in sweet potatoes, cantaloupe melon, carrots and dark leafy greens, such as kale and spinach.

Ellagic acid is another potent polyphenol, which has antioxidant and anti-inflammatory properties. It has also been reported to reduce the risk of cancer. The best food source is raspberries. Other good food sources: strawberries, blackberries, grapes, walnuts and pecans.

Resveratrol is my favourite polyphenol, and is found predominantly in the skin of grapes and red wine! Resveratrol promotes cardiovascular health and also cognitive health. Good food sources: blueberries, strawberries, dark chocolate and peanuts.

Micronutrient	Vitamin A	Vitamin C	Vitamin D	Vitamin E	Zinc	Selenium
Men	0.7mg	40mg	10mcg	4mg	9.5mg	75mcg
Women	0.6mg	40mg	10mcg	3mg	7mg	60mcg

Flavonoids are also part of the polyphenol class of phytonutrients, and are rich in antioxidant, anti-inflammatory and antimicrobial properties. Also in the flavonoid family we have flavones, anthocyanins, flavanones, isoflavones and flavonols. Good food sources: apples, onions, soy, coffee, legumes, ginger and green tea.

Glucosinolates are sulfur-containing compounds that may promote longevity by protecting against chronic disease. Good food sources: broccoli, cauliflower, cabbage, mustard and horseradish.

Variety is the spice of life

Herbs and spices are also high in phytochemicals, and including them in your daily diet not only benefits your immunity and health, but also provides excitement to food. I always advise clients to cook with herbs and spices regularly and – if possible – to use several at a time. Rich in phytochemicals, herbs and spices can help to combat harmful inflammation and promote good health. I use a lot of different herbs and spices in the recipes in Part 3, so let's take a look at some of the main players:

Turmeric – this spice gets a lot of press. It's a good source of curcumin, an antioxidant that eases inflammation, and studies also indicate that curcumin may help ease pain. In addition, further studies have demonstrated that frequently consuming even small amounts of turmeric may help prevent or slow down Alzheimer's disease. It has also been shown to protect gut lining and inhibit the growth of harmful pathogens.

Cardamom – this is a sweet and pungent spice that has been reported to help combat inflammation. In addition, out of all the spices, cardamom is a great source of immunity-nourishing zinc.

Chilli pepper – this will certainly give your food a kick, which is down to capsaicin, the compound that makes chillies spicy. Chilli may also boost your metabolism and help maintain blood-vessel health.

Cinnamon – sweet and ultra-versatile, you can add it to so many different dishes. I use it a lot in porridge (oatmeal), baking, and main dishes such as curries. Research has shown that cinnamon may also help combat inflammation and oxidative stress, as well as helping to protect against harmful bacteria.

Ginger – anti-inflammatory with antioxidant properties, ginger can soothe the digestive tract and gut lining. Studies also show that ginger has anti-inflammatory and antioxidant properties, and may play a role in preventing diseases like cancer.

Rosemary – this is a beautiful and fragrant herb that is very rich in antioxidants, which prevent cell damage and protect against damaging free radicals.

Cocoa – a spice with many health benefits, the cocoa bean is loaded with flavonoids, which we know are ultra-powerful phytochemicals.

Garlic – a food that I include in my cooking almost every day, which has been used for centuries as both an ingredient and a medicine. Eating garlic offers numerous health benefits, including supporting strong immunity, as it contains compounds that help our immune system fight harmful pathogens. Whole fresh garlic contains alliin, but when garlic is chopped or crushed this converts to allicin, which isn't stable, so quickly converts to other compounds that are said to give garlic its medicinal properties. Additionally, as a potent antibiotic, garlic has been shown to combat strains of *Staphylococcus*, the bacteria associated with staph infections. Tips for cooking with garlic:

- Crush or chop/slice all your garlic before you eat it (this increases the allicin content).

- Before you cook with crushed garlic, let it stand for 10 minutes before cooking (this helps prevent the loss of its beneficial properties).

- Use a lot of garlic, ideally more than one clove per meal, if possible.

chapter 8:
can intermittent fasting help immunity?

Humans have been fasting for thousands of years in the name of religion, and fasting has now become very popular for lifestyle reasons in the Western world in the last decade. There are different forms of intermittent fasting (IF), but it generally refers to eating between 0 and 30 per cent of normal daily energy intake. IF regimens can be categorized into fasting for up to 24 hours once or twice a week, with ad libitum food intake for the remaining days, known as periodic prolonged fasting (PF); eating for 8 hours then fasting for the other 16 hours of the day (time-restricted feeding or TRF); and alternating between feasting and fast days (alternate-day fasting or ADF).

IF refers to the umbrella term which includes the different intermittent fasting protocols.

PF refers to periodic fasting (whole-day fasting is an example of this).

TRF refers to time-restricted feeding (16:8 is an example of this) – it is also known as 'time-restricted eating'.

ADF refers to alternate-day fasting (the 5:2 is similar to this, but only involves two fasting days).

Increasing studies in both animal and human models have shown that IF is effective for weight loss, and reducing insulin resistance, blood pressure, cholesterol, oxidative damage and inflammation. More recently, IF has been shown to also benefit our gut microbiome.

Fasting and our gut bacteria

While the field is still in its infancy, an emerging body of evidence suggests beneficial effects of fasting on the health of the gut through increasing the microbial diversity, abundance and resilience, with possible clinical implications related to improving immunity. The major bacteria that loves fasting is called *Akkermansia*. This bacteria thrives when you fast, feeding off your gut lining and cleaning it, which has been shown to increase the diversity of the other bacterial species. Nonetheless, again it is about balance, as too long a time without eating and *Akkermansia* has been reported to damage the gut lining.

In a 2015 study, the researchers allocated 13 men and women who were all overweight to a diet where they consumed 600–800 calories a day for one week[77]. Stool samples of the participants showed increased bacterial diversity and a significant increase in *Akkermansia* and also another beneficial bacteria, *Bifidobacterium*. At present, there are a limited number of small-scale human studies that consider the role of *Akkermansia*. However, in a pilot study[78] of nine people during the month of Ramadan, that involved 17 hours of fasting a day, results indicated an increase of the 'good' bacteria, including *Akkermansia*. In a second study by the same researchers, it was determined that fasting led to changes in the composition of the gut microbiota, including microbial richness[79].

Like us, our gut bacteria also function on a daily rhythm – their powerful circadian rhythm is key for our immunity, and is enhanced by fasting.

While current research is still in its infancy, findings of the current human studies suggest that intermittent fasting may play a potentially beneficial role in altering the gut microbiota, leading to enhanced changes in microbiota composition and diversity. However, it should be noted that the present studies have small sample sizes, therefore larger clinical trials with longer observation timeframes are needed.

Fasting and our immunity

Animal studies show that fasting has the potential to reduce the severity of many autoimmune diseases. In a 2014 study, it was demonstrated that fasting cycles of three days actually reversed the autoimmunity in a group of mice by killing damaged immune cells, generating new cells, and turning on progenitor cells (cells similar to stem cells), which can regenerate damaged nerves[80]. In addition, the researchers reported that fasting is particularly effective in killing off old immune cells that have lost the ability to distinguish between the cells of its own body and invaders such as viruses and bacteria.

Furthermore, a 2017 review, which looked at the existing research, reported that relatively long-term fasting, or fasting cycles followed by refeeding, appear to reduce the biological rate of ageing and promote anti-inflammatory effects[81]. The authors concluded that this, in turn, may contribute to easing and potentially reversing a number of autoimmune conditions, as well as immunosenescence, by killing the damaged cells and replacing them with younger, more efficient cells. Thus, fasting *could* repair an impaired immune system, and may have the potential to treat autoimmune conditions. However, further clinical research is needed to establish the precise role of fasting on the immune system.

Want to try IF?

If you are new to fasting and keen to give it a go, I suggest starting with time-restricted feeding (TRF), where you fast for 16 hours and eat in an 8-hour window. I have followed this fasting protocol for over 15 years, and consume no food from 7pm overnight to 11am the following day. You are able to drink water, herbal teas and black coffee during the fasting period. If you can't do the full 16 hours initially, just work up to it, like I did. Start by fasting for 12 hours (say, 7pm–7am), then build to 14 hours (7pm–9am), and then the full 16 hours (7pm–11am).

Another popular protocol is the 5:2 method, where for two days of the week you consume 600–800 calories. Some days you may need to eat in the 14-hour window, and this is absolutely fine – let it work for you and your lifestyle. It is important when you are fasting to preserve fat-free muscle mass (FFM), which can be achieved through weight-bearing exercise. It is crucial that you ensure you consume a nutrient-dense diet, as studies have shown that eating a dramatically restricted diet may cause the immune system to deteriorate. Also, if you do decide to give intermittent fasting a go, be aware of any changes in thyroid function or hormonal alterations.

Maintaining a healthy weight is vital for reducing your risk of inflammation, and intermittent fasting can be very effective for weight loss. Top tips for weight management:

- Give time-restricted feeding, such as the 16:8 a go. Start by fasting for 12 hours (7pm–7am). As you get used to this regime, try and go another hour (7pm–8am), until you can manage the 16 hours (7pm–11am).

- Ensure a good-quality protein in every meal – free-range eggs, wild salmon, soybeans.

- Eat more vegetables in place of white refined carbs, such as white pasta, white bread and white rice.

- Eat at least two portions of fatty fish a week – wild salmon, sardines, trout, mackerel.

- Limit all refined-sugar and processed foods, and if you do have sweet-craving, opt for 70 per cent cocoa solids.

- Aim for 30 minutes of moderate-intensity exercise every day, such as fast walking, cycling or swimming.

chapter 9:
how exercise benefits your immune system

Exercise is beneficial for both our immunity and gut health. Research in humans has confirmed that exercise increases microbial diversity, and has been shown to decrease inflammation and infection, while promoting recovery and enhancing immune function[82].

Exercise and the gut

Our gut bacteria play a role in how physical activity can decrease our risk of disease, but the mechanism is not yet fully known. However, exercise has been shown to promote the immune system in positive ways, then, in turn, the immune system sends chemical signals to the gut bacteria[83]. In addition, physical activity itself can directly affect the composition of the gut bacteria. The short-chain fatty acid, butyrate, is made by our gut bacteria and is very important for our immunity – exercise encourages our bacteria to make more of it[84].

In a study from the University of Illinois, researchers found that exercising for just six weeks could impact the gut microbiome. The study participants were assigned an exercise programme consisting of cardiovascular exercises for 30–60 minutes, three times a week for six weeks. At the end of the study, the researchers sampled the participants' gut microbiomes, and discovered that the microbiomes had changed. Some participants experienced an increase in certain gut microbes and others a decrease. Many had an increase in microbes that are involved in the production of beneficial short-chain fatty acids, such as our friend butyrate. After the initial period of six weeks, the participants then returned to six weeks of their normal inactive lifestyle. When the researchers sampled participants' microbiomes again at the end of this sedentary period, they found the microbiomes had returned to how they were before the period of exercise. This suggests the impact of exercise on the microbiome may be short-lived, hence it appears that exercise needs to be performed regularly.

When it comes to exercise, just as in our diets, we need balance, since too much exercise has been shown to result in temporary gut damage and impaired gut function[85]. This appears to be caused by an increase in body temperature and decreased blood flow. However, physical activity is imperative for health and for the lymphatic system. We need to keep the super-important and immunity-nourishing lymph moving as it contains a significant proportion of our immune cells. As we know, ageing decreases our immune function, and the thymus gland, which produces our T cells, shrinks. However, exercise is one of the most effective strategies when it comes to strengthening immunity, as putting your muscles through their paces, promotes the release of a hormone (IL-7), which helps prevent thymic involution so our thymus can continue to make our important T cells.

In the last few decades, numerous studies have investigated how exercise impacts immunity, and it is commonly acknowledged that regular moderate-intensity exercise has a positive effect on immunity. One study found that 30 minutes of brisk walking increased the circulation of NK cells and white blood cells, and when these immune cells come face to face with a harmful pathogen, they are able to kill it effectively[86]. However, the researchers reported that about three hours after exercise immune cells head back to the tissues they derived from. So it appears that the immune-supporting effects of exercise may be somewhat short-lived, which is why the 'regular' part of regular exercise is so important.

Furthermore, regular physical activity, in the long term, has been shown to delay the changes that occur to the ageing immune system, thereby decreasing the infection risk. A recent 2020 analysis, published in the international journal *Exercise Immunology Review*, assessed the effect of exercise on our immune function and investigated whether the immune system is impacted positively or negatively after exercise. The analysis determined that, rather than the act of exercising itself, infections are more likely to be associated with poor nutrition, inadequate sleep, stress, travel and, significantly, exposure to pathogens at large events such as marathons[87].

What exercise is most effective?

For overall health, UK government guidelines recommend that adults aged 19–64 should aim to be active daily. Over a week, activity should add up to at least 150 minutes of moderate-intensity exercise, such as brisk walking, swimming or cycling[88]. Alternatively, comparable benefits can be achieved through 75 minutes of vigorous-intensity activity, such as running, swimming or HIIT, spread across the week. However, 75 minutes or more of intense exercise may be too much for some people, as when you go that long at a high intensity, stress hormones such as cortisol increase, and the immune system does not respond well to that.

Adults should also undertake physical activity to improve muscle strength on at least two days a week. This is particularly important if you practise intermittent fasting. Good examples of this type of activity include weight lifting, yoga, Pilates – or any activity which involves you using body weight or working against a

resistance. Even carrying heavy food shopping can be beneficial.

US recommendations as to how much exercise one should be doing per week are similar, with the advice that adults should be performing at least 150 minutes of moderate-intensity aerobic exercise a week, as well as two muscle-strengthening exercise sessions.

> - In England, 1 in 4 women and 1 in 5 men are classed as physically inactive – doing less than 30 minutes of moderate physical activity per week.
>
> - In addition, only 34 per cent of men and 24 per cent of women undertake muscle-strengthening activities at least twice a week.

In a study of 150 adults, aged 50 and over, moderate physical activity was shown to significantly reduce the risk of contracting an acute respiratory infection, such as cold or flu. The researchers also showed that severity of an infection was also reduced[89]. Moderate-intensity aerobic exercise, such as walking or cycling, for 30–60 minutes a day appears to be the most effective when it comes to optimizing immune function.

I personally love walking – it is what we were built to do. My great-grandmother lived to 106 and walked at least two miles every day until she was in her late nineties. A 30-minute walk in the fresh air decreases the duration and severity of a mild infection, while stimulating the lymph to do its job properly, in addition to supporting gut health and immunity. It is also a fantastic stress buster, and successful stress management, as we will see in the next chapter, is essential when striving for a balanced immune system.

chapter 10:
how to manage stress effectively

Stress and the immune system

Stress can have a significant impact on both your mental and physical health, impacting immunity, and putting us at a greater risk of infection and disease. If you have been experiencing intense stress for a lengthy period, you may well be chronically stressed, putting you at a greater risk for developing autoimmune conditions.

In the early 1980s, researchers from the Ohio State University College of Medicine were intrigued by animal studies associating stress with infection, and for a decade they studied medical students and found that the students' immunity decreased every year due to the stress of a three-day exam period[90]. In addition, they noted that the students had fewer NK cells, which fight viral infections and tumours, and nearly stopped producing interferon, a cytokine that is crucial to innate and adaptive immunity.

Furthermore, a different team of researchers analyzed 300 studies on stress and health[91] and detected interesting patterns. Studies that stressed people for a few minutes discovered a burst of one type of 'first responder' activity mixed with other signs of weakening. However, for recurrent and chronic stress of any prolonged period (from a few days to a few months or years), all aspects of immunity were adversely affected. In addition, the research showed that the participants who were already unwell or elderly were more susceptible to stress-associated immunity changes.

Mind:body interaction

Managing chronic stress can help us to fight germs and strengthen our immunity. This was confirmed by researchers who compared the immune function of exam-stressed medical students given hypnosis and relaxation training with that of students without training. At first, the immune responses of the two groups both seemed to decrease; however, closer review highlighted that some of the students took this exercise more seriously than others. The students that were committed and consistent in their practice, did have significantly superior immune function during the exams than those who did not do the relaxation exercises, or performed them only intermittently.

Mind:body interaction is key. Research has shown that chronic feelings of loneliness can help to predict health status, maybe since lonely people experience greater psychological stress, or perhaps experience it more intensely. That stress then dampens down immunity and hampers the body's ability to fight infection. Studies have confirmed the value of good friends, and even a few close friends have been shown to help someone feel connected and able to deal with stressful events. In fact, the presence of friends can make us view stress differently, as one study demonstrated[92]. The researchers asked participants who were either alone or with a friend to estimate the steepness of a hill in front of them. With no support close by, the participants who were on their own perceived the hill as steeper than the subjects who were accompanied by a friend.

Stress and the gut

Stress not only ravages our immunity, but it also wreaks havoc with our gut health, and it's increasingly recognized that stress changes our gut microbiota community structure and also activity[93]. In fact, it may be one causal factor in dysbiosis[94]. Furthermore, psychological stress has also been associated with multiple GI disorders[95]. We don't fully know why yet, but the association appears to be attributed to stress-induced alterations in communication between the gut and the brain (the gut-brain axis), to include altered signalling along the vagus nerve and enteric nervous system; and HPA-axis activation resulting in immunomodulation, inflammation, intestinal damage, and increased GI permeability[91]. All of these factors have the potential to adversely impact the gut microbiota and our gut health.

In a mouse study, the researchers investigated how stress-induced alterations to the gut microbiome influence health. They observed that sharing a cage with more aggressive mice, which is considered a 'social disruption' stressor, decreased 'good' bacteria, reduced the overall diversity of the gut microbiome, and encouraged harmful bacteria to multiply. This resulted in the animals becoming more vulnerable to infection and having gut inflammation. In a follow-up study, the researchers found that administering mice broad-spectrum antibiotics to suppress gut bacteria inhibited stress-induced inflammation. Likewise, they reported that germ-free mice also didn't show stress-induced inflammation, but when the germ-free mice were colonized with a normal population of bacteria, stress once again resulted in gut inflammation[96].

Stress-induced changes to the microbiome may also affect the brain and behaviour. A study conducted by Harvard Medical School reported that elite-level athletes who stayed calm during stressful sports competitions shared common gut microbiome traits, suggesting that there might well be an association between mental resilience and the gut microbiome.

How to manage stress

There are several scientifically proven strategies for managing stress, including exercise, yoga, meditation, mindfulness, and by having healthy, positive friendships.

Regular exercise

We know exercise is good for us on so many different levels, including promoting gut and immune health, as we saw in the last chapter. However, exercise is also an excellent 'de-stressor', and many people experience an immediate boost to their mood after exercise. Fortunately, those positive feelings don't end there, but generally increase over time. So you are very likely to notice increased feelings of well-being if you commit to a regular exercise regimen. As well as reducing stress, regular physical activity benefits health in numerous other ways, which may indirectly help to reduce your stress levels. Exercise is also an effective way to help you sleep better at night.

Yoga

The word 'yoga' comes from the Sanskrit word 'yuji', meaning yoke or union, and the practice of yoga unites mind and body. Yoga has been shown to modulate the stress response system, thereby reducing blood pressure, decreasing heart rate and regulating breathing. Several studies have highlighted that practising yoga can reduce cortisol levels, which we know produce many of the harmful effects of stress. One study demonstrated the impressive effect of yoga on stress by assessing 24 women who defined themselves as emotionally distressed. After a 12-week yoga programme, the women had significantly decreased cortisol levels. They also reported reduced stress, anxiety, fatigue and depression[97]. A later study of 131 people had similar results, showing that 10 weeks of yoga helped to reduce stress and anxiety, while also improving quality of life and mental health[98].

A small study conducted by the University of Utah provided some insight into the impact of yoga on the stress response by looking at individuals' responses to pain. The researchers observed that people who had a poorly regulated response to stress were also more sensitive to pain. Their subjects were 12 experienced yoga practitioners, 14 people with fibromyalgia (a condition thought to be stress-related and characterized by hypersensitivity to pain) and 16 healthy volunteers. When the three groups were subjected to more or less painful thumbnail pressure, the participants with fibromyalgia reported pain at lower pressure levels compared with the other subjects. Magnetic resonance imaging (MRI) showed they also had the greatest activity in areas of the brain associated with the pain response. In contrast, the yoga practitioners had the greatest pain tolerance and lowest pain-related brain activity during the MRI. The study highlights the value of stress-management techniques, which can help a person manage their stress and also pain responses.

Meditation

Another strategy that has been proven to be effective at reducing stress is meditation. A study of nearly 1,300 adults demonstrated that meditation may decrease stress. Notably, this effect was strongest in individuals with the highest levels of stress[99]. Studies have also reported that practising meditation may alleviate symptoms of conditions associated with stress, such as IBS. Furthermore, meditation has also been reported to be helpful for strengthening our immunity. Research has been shown that it can promote the functioning and number of T cells and NK cells, decrease the incidence of illness, and improve a person's health and quality of life[100].

Mindfulness

Mindfulness is a state of intentional, non-judgemental focus on the present moment. In a review of meditation studies[101], the authors reported solid evidence that individuals who had mindfulness-based therapy during times of stress, were less prone to respond pessimistically. They also demonstrated that people who participated in mindfulness-based therapy or mindfulness-based stress reduction were more able to focus on the present and less likely to worry and to think about a negative thought or experience repeatedly. It is hypothesized that the beneficial effects of mindfulness are linked to its capacity to reduce the body's stress response. We know that chronic stress can impair immunity, and contribute to the worsening of many other health problems. However, by reducing the stress response, mindfulness may have other beneficial effects throughout the body, including strengthening immunity.

Key points

· Avoid prolonged chronic stress.

· Adopt stress-management techniques that work for you – going for a walk, yoga, meditation or practising mindfulness.

· Spend time with friends and laugh – laughter really is the best medicine!

As well as affecting your immunity and gut health, chronic stress can also lead to sleep problems. Stress and sleep go hand in hand, as we will discover in the next chapter.

chapter 11:
the significance of sleep and your immune system

For over 2,000 years, the relationship between immunity and sleep has been a hot topic, and even Hippocrates confirmed the role of 'sleepiness' during an acute infection[102].

Along with the circadian rhythm, sleep is known to regulate immune function. Ensuring you get sufficient sleep is crucial for gut health and immunity, since numerous studies have shown a significant decrease in immunity, after either a night without sleep or after a lengthy continual period of sleep deprivation[103]. The studies' findings confirm that both lymphocytes and NK cells are reduced when we are sleep-deprived and immune function is altered. In fact, one study showed that just a single night with a lack of sleep can decrease NK cell activity by as much as 30 per cent. A second study also reported a reduction of 30 per cent in NK cell activity in healthy participants who slept less than seven hours compared with participants who slept seven to nine hours[104].

Chronic disturbance of our circadian rhythm and sleep deprivation, which impacts our gut bacteria and promotes alterations in their composition, is also associated with dysbiosis. These harmful changes may then lead to inflammation, metabolic disorders and weakened immunity. This process may also alter the metabolism of neurotransmitters and result in nervous system dysfunction. The individual then experiences sleep problems and this, ultimately, initiates a vicious cycle. However, research shows that individuals who get morning sunlight exposure reportedly have a better quality of sleep. Further studies have also highlighted that vitamin D impacts sleep quality, and low serum levels of vitamin D have been linked to a greater risk of sleep disorders and inferior sleep quality[105]. Ensuring we get enough natural sunlight is key for a good night's sleep.

Sleep deprivation may also increase inflammation and stress hormones in your body, and this may explain why not getting enough sleep is linked with worse gut symptoms. Therefore, ensuring sufficient good-quality sleep is key for our immunity, gut health and overall health.

Let's explore some of the most effective strategies for ensuring sufficient shut-eye.

How to sleep well

Sleep requirements differ from person to person; however, the NHS states that most healthy adults need between seven and nine hours of sleep each night to allow our bodies to recover and function at their best, while children and teens need even more[106]. It is commonly believed that our sleep requirements reduce as we get older; however, elderly individuals still need at least seven hours of sleep. Unfortunately, many of us aren't sleeping as much as we should. Of the 5,000 individuals who participated in a British Sleep Council survey, 74 per cent said they had less than seven hours sleep a night, while 12 per cent confessed they had less than five hours, which is more than the 7 per cent who said the same in 2013.

If you are struggling with your sleep, consider the following tips:

During the day

- Try to wake up at the same time each day.

- Aim to go for a walk before breakfast, as morning light turns off your brain's production of melatonin, the hormone that encourages sleep.

- Try to get outside in the sunshine at some point during the day, as this will help keep your vitamin D levels topped up (studies have shown that low vitamin D levels are associated with inferior quality and decreased duration of sleep). It also helps to maintain your body's circadian rhythms, which impacts your sleep-wake cycle.

- Exercise regularly, but try to exercise at least a few hours before you go to bed. Exercising too close to bedtime can make it harder to fall asleep and also lead to disrupted sleep.

- Limit caffeine from midday. Caffeine increases the stress hormone, cortisol, which can not only impact sleep, but increased levels may also reduce your immune system's ability to fight infection.

- Avoid lengthy afternoon naps.

- Stress is an important cause of insomnia, so adopt the most appropriate stress-management for you.

Before bed

- Refrain from eating late at night. If your gut is having to do a lot of substantial digestion work, this will impact the quality of your sleep and make it harder to fall asleep.

- Limit alcohol and nicotine in the evening, as they can interrupt your sleep.

- Adopt a relaxing routine before bedtime, such as listening to soothing music or having a warm scented-oil bath. Try an Epsom salt (magnesium salt) bath, which has been shown to promote sleep.

- Write down three positive things that occurred that day. This is part of my bedtime routine. In fact, this has been shown to be one of the most effective strategies to boost mood.

- At least 30 minutes before bed, turn off your electronic devices – light from these devices can stimulate brain activity, making it more difficult to fall asleep.

- Dim the lights before bedtime, as this will encourage your brain to realize that it's time for bed.

- Create a relaxing environment in your bedroom – studies have indicated that there is a strong association in people's minds between sleep and the bedroom.

- Make sure your bedroom isn't too hot or cold – 18.3°C (65°F) has been suggested as an ideal sleeping temperature.

In bed
- Avoid using your phone or laptop; instead read a book to help you relax.

- Focus on steady breathing to help you relax.

- If you are unable to fall asleep, read a book or listen to music until you are ready to go to sleep.

Glycine

Glycine is an amino acid that has been shown to help regulate the body's immune response, limit inflammation, and promote healing and repair. It also helps the body make serotonin, which is a neurotransmitter that has a profound impact on sleep and also mood. Glycine affects sleep in different ways, and several studies indicate that supplementation of 3g of glycine before bedtime can improve sleep quality, and reduce sleepiness and fatigue during the day in sleep deprived individuals[107]. Glycine supplementation before bedtime has also been reported to help you fall asleep quicker, reduce insomnia symptoms and promote sleep efficiency.

Do note that there are commonly used medications that may interact with glycine. If you take any medication or supplements, please do seek advice from your doctor before beginning to use glycine as a supplement. Clozapine is one drug that is used in the treatment of schizophrenia, and supplementing with glycine whilst taking clozapine may decrease the effectiveness of clozapine. Thus, it is recommended that people who are taking clozapine do not use glycine. Also, women who are pregnant or breastfeeding should not supplement with glycine, since we don't know if it's safe to use during pregnancy or lactation.

Key points
- Keep to a consistent bedtime routine in a dark environment.

- Avoid screen time before bedtime.

- Aim for 7–9 hours sleep time.

- Keep to a consistent waking time.

- Aim for a walk in the morning.

- Ensure you get some sunshine during the day.

- Avoid caffeine-containing drinks or foods after 12pm.

- Limit alcohol as it is known to disturb sleep.

- Supplement with 3g of glycine, if advised.

chapter 12:
the power of light

Sunlight is essential for many important bodily functions, including maintaining your circadian rhythm, mood and for producing vitamin D. In Chapter 7, we learned how vital vitamin D is for strong and balanced immunity, since it is involved in a vast array of immune-system activities. Vitamin D has also been reported to regulate gene expression and further exert its immunomodulatory effects on immune cells[108]. Also, in the skin, there are cells known as keratinocytes, which make a potent immune-nourishing substance known as interleukin-1 (IL-1), which promote the number of T cells by helping them to multiply rapidly. Natural sunlight stimulates IL-1, which is another reason why it is important we get enough sunshine.

While sunlight allows us to make vitamin D, a surprise research finding reported another significant benefit of getting some sunshine. Scientists at Georgetown University in the US, observed that sunlight, through a different mechanism to the manufacturing of vitamin D, 'energizes' T cells, which we know play a crucial role in our immunity[109]. T cells need to move quickly to carry out their function and get to the infection site. The researchers discovered that low levels of blue light in the sun's rays allows T cells to move quicker, confirming that sunlight directly activates our important immune cells, by enhancing their movement.

Studies have shown that autoimmune diseases tend to share a predisposition for vitamin D deficiency, which negatively alters the gut microbiome and the integrity of the gut barrier[110]. Low vitamin D appears to increase the permeability of the gut barrier and heighten immune activity – remember our goal is balanced immune activity. This, in turn, alters microbial composition and the ability of our microbes to move across the gut barrier, leading to negative interaction with the immune system. However, fortunately, researchers have reported that the composition of the gut microbiome can be positively impacted by vitamin D status and exposure[111]. Further, scientists have confirmed that it is clear that the immune system and microbiome are very closely connected, and that vitamin D is a key mediator in this dynamic[110].

Vitamin D deficiency

Vitamin D deficiency is a global health problem caused mainly by insufficient exposure to sunlight, and it is estimated that about 1 billion people globally have low levels of the vitamin in their blood[112]. According to a 2011 study, 41.6 per cent of adults in the US are deficient[113]. However, many people are unaware that they may even have such a deficiency. For most people, exposing your arms and face for 10–15 minutes a few times a week and eating oily, fatty fish twice a week, is sufficient to maintain your vitamin D levels.

To supplement or not

Taking a vitamin D supplement in winter may be recommended for some individuals, especially if a blood check highlights you are deficient. If you do decide to supplement, just be cautious, as it is possible to take too much vitamin D, particularly if you take a high-dose supplement, and/or for a prolonged duration. This can result in a build-up of calcium in the body, which can damage your bones, heart and kidneys. If you suspect a vitamin D deficiency, I would suggest speaking with your medical practitioner who may advise you to have a blood test to check your levels. Once you know for sure you need to supplement, you can go from there, as too much can be as detrimental as too little – we are aiming for balance.

chapter 13: putting it all together

Our fast-paced and modern lifestyles tend to stress our gut microbiomes and immune systems rather than helping to support them. By making the right nutrition choices, exercising appropriately, managing stress, ensuring optimal sleep and sufficient sunshine exposure, we can achieve strong and balanced gut health and immunity. Food choice is one of the greatest opportunities to improve your immunity and health – it is all in your control.

The Immunity Plan

This is an easy go-to table that summarizes all the guidance in the book (recommendations are based on UK government daily dietary guidelines for adults aged 18-64).

	How much	Food sources
Energy (kcal/day)	2500 (men) / 2000 (women)	
Macronutrients		
Carbs	333g (men) / 267g (women) 30g fibre (men and women)	Vegetables, fruits, wholegrains, legumes, nuts and seeds.
Protein	56g (men) / 45g (women)	Meat, poultry, fish, eggs, dairy products, soy, nuts and seeds.
Fats (less than) Saturated Fat Monounsaturated Fat Polyunsaturated Fat Omega 3	97g (men) / 78g (women) 31g (men) / 24g (women) 36g (men) / 29g (women) 18g (men) / 14g (women) 2 portions of fatty fish a week (men and women)	Focus on the 'healthy' fats found in foods such as avocado, olive oil, nuts such as walnuts, seeds such as flax seeds (linseeds), fatty fish such as wild salmon, mackerel, sardines and trout.
Salt	6g or less a day (men and women)	Natural food sources include meat, seafood and eggs. It is also found in a lot of processed foods, such as bread, so do read the labels carefully.

	How much	Food sources
Micronutrients		
Vitamin A	0.7mg (men) / 0.6mg (women)	Liver, full-fat (whole) milk and cheese are dietary sources of retinol ('pre-formed' vitamin A). Dark green leafy vegetables and orange-coloured fruits and vegetables, e.g. carrots, sweet potato, butternut squash, cantaloupe melon and papaya, are dietary sources of carotenoids, which can be converted to vitamin A by the body.
Vitamin C	40mg (men and women)	Citrus fruits, blackcurrants, strawberries, papaya, kiwi, green vegetables, (bell) peppers and tomatoes.
Vitamin D	10mcg (men and women)	Oily fish, eggs, fortified breakfast cereals, fortified spreads and fortified dairy products, and some mushrooms.
Vitamin E	4mg (men) / 3mg (women)	Wheat germ, nuts, seeds, avocado and spinach.
Selenium	75mcg (men) / 60mcg (women)	Nuts and seeds (for example Brazil nuts, cashews and sunflower seeds), eggs, offal (variety meats), poultry, fish and shellfish.
Zinc	9.5mg (men) / 7mg (women)	Meat, poultry, cheese, shellfish (including crab and mussels), nuts and seeds (in particular pumpkin seeds and pine nuts), wholegrain breakfast cereals and wholegrain and seeded breads.
Other nutrients		
Prebiotics	N/A	Jerusalem artichokes, chicory (endive), apples, bananas, cauliflower, garlic, leeks, onions, black beans, butter (lima) beans, chickpeas (garbanzo beans) and camomile tea.
Probiotics	N/A	Fermented foods such as sauerkraut, kimchi, kefir and natural live yoghurt.

Lifestyle	How much	Examples
Exercise	30 minutes moderate activity every day (if possible).	Walking, swimming, cycling and dancing.
Sleep	7–9 hours per night.	(If you are recovering from an infection or undergoing significant stress you will potentially need more.)
Sunlight	10–15 minutes of exposure several times a week – ensure your face and arms are exposed, if possible.	Try to get out in the sunshine for a walk during the morning.
Stress Management	Adopt the most appropriate stress management technique for you.	Exercise, yoga, mindfulness practice, meditation, catching up with friends and laughing!

Appendix I

Micronutrients and their role in our immune systems

Nutrient	Role
Vitamin A	Helps support T cells (a type of white blood cell that helps identify pathogens).
Vitamin C	Helps immune cells attack pathogens, helps get rid of immune cells from the site of infection; also helps to maintain the skin, which is our external barrier to infection.
Vitamin D	Has numerous effects on immune system cells, and low status is associated with reduced immune response.
Vitamin E	This antioxidant is important for the normal function of the immune cells.
Selenium	Helps produce new immune cells and can help to strengthen response to infection.
Zinc	Helps produce new immune cells; also encourages the development of NK cells that help to combat viruses. Zinc also supports the communication between our different immune cells.

Adapted from British Nutrition Foundation, 2020

Appendix II

Phytonutrient-rich foods featured in the recipes

Foods	Phytonutrients
Apples	Catechins, flavonols and tartaric acid
Artichokes	Carotenoids
Beetroot (beets)	Carotenoids
Berries	Anthocyanins and anthocyanidins, lignans and tannic acid
Broccoli (also Brussels sprouts, cabbage, cauliflower and kale)	Allylic sulfides, carotenoids, lignans and vitamin C
Cantaloupe melon	Carotenoids
Carrots	Carotenoids and lignins
Chilli peppers	Capsaicin
Cocoa and dark chocolate	Flavonols and catechins
Flax seeds (linseeds) and oil seeds	Lignans
Garlic	Limonene, flavonols and allylic sulfides
Legumes	Catechins, carotenoids, flavonols, lignans, omega fatty acids and saponins
Nuts and seeds	Phytic acid, phytosterols and stilbenes (resveratrol)
Olive oil	Hydroxytyrosol, oleuropein and oleocanthal
Onions	Flavonols and allylic sulfides
Pumpkin	Carotenoids and lignans
Red cabbage	Anthocyanins and anthocyanidins
Red grapes (and wine)	Catechins, ellagic acid, flavonols and stilbenes (resveratrol)
Soy	Isoflavones, phytic acid, phytosterols and saponins
Spinach	Carotenoids and lignins
Squash and sweet potatoes	Carotenoids
Tomatoes	Carotenoids and vitamin C
Whole grains	Lignins, organo or allylic sulfides and saponins
(Bell) Peppers	Carotenoids and vitamin C

part three:
the recipes

Recipe notes:
All eggs are medium unless otherwise
specified. I recommend using free-range
or organic eggs whenever possible.

The oven temperatures given are for
conventional ovens. If your oven is fan-assisted
(convection), lower the temperature by
10–20°C.

<u>df</u>   dairy-free

<u>gf</u>   gluten-free

<u>vg</u>   vegan

Sample meal planners

Breakfast can be omitted if you choose to fast or eaten later as brunch.

	Breakfast	Lunch	Dinner
Monday	Baked Eggs in Avocado (p.79)	Roasted Pepper and Tomato Soup (p.86)	Hearty Chicken Casserole (p.169)
Tuesday	Figgy Apple and Cinnamon Porridge (p.70) with a handful of berries	Chicken, Broccoli and Beetroot Salad (p.92)	Pea and Lemon Risotto (p.150)
Wednesday	Turmeric Scramble (p.77)	Wild Salmon Veggie Bowl (p.122)	Pumpkin and Spinach Curry (p.181)
Thursday	The Immunity Smoothie (p.67)	Chickpea and Cumin Burgers (p.113)	Salmon Fish Cakes with Garlic Aïoli (p.146)
Friday	Nutty Maple Granola (p.72)	Tuna, Fennel and Bean Salad (p.101)	Veggie Cottage Pie with Sweet Potato Mash (p.135)
Saturday	Banana and Almond Breakfast Pot (p.67)	Kale and Goat's Cheese Frittata (p.103)	Aubergine and Tomato Hake (p.130)
Sunday	Overnight Chocolate Oats (p.71)	Avocado and Black Bean Eggs (p.109)	King Prawn Jalfrezi (p.183) with wholegrain rice or Cauliflower Rice (p.192)

	Breakfast	Lunch	Dinner
Monday	No-Flour Banana Pancakes (p.70)	Sundried Tomato, Feta and Basil Omelette (p.104)	Chicken Banana Korma (p.173)
Tuesday	Poached Egg and Mushroom Hash (p.75)	Chicken and Vegetable Soup (p.82)	Chickpea and Bean Chilli (p.143)
Wednesday	The Immunity Smoothie (p.67)	Zingy Teriyaki Salmon Salad (p.95)	Red Lentil and Rosemary Patties (p.163)
Thursday	Raspberry Chia Bowl (p.68)	Broccoli and Turmeric Hash (p.111)	Fruity Lamb Tagine (p.160)
Friday	Nutty Maple Granola (p.72)	Beetroot, Spinach and Goat's Cheese Couscous (p.120)	Easy Peasy Paella (p.139)
Saturday	Poached Eggs with Spinach and Walnuts (p.76)	Satay Tofu Skewers (p.116)	Broccoli Lemon Chicken with Cashews (p.164)
Sunday	Portobello Mushrooms with Kale and Feta (p.74)	Turkey Burgers (p.115)	Puy Lentils with Smoked Tofu (p.170)

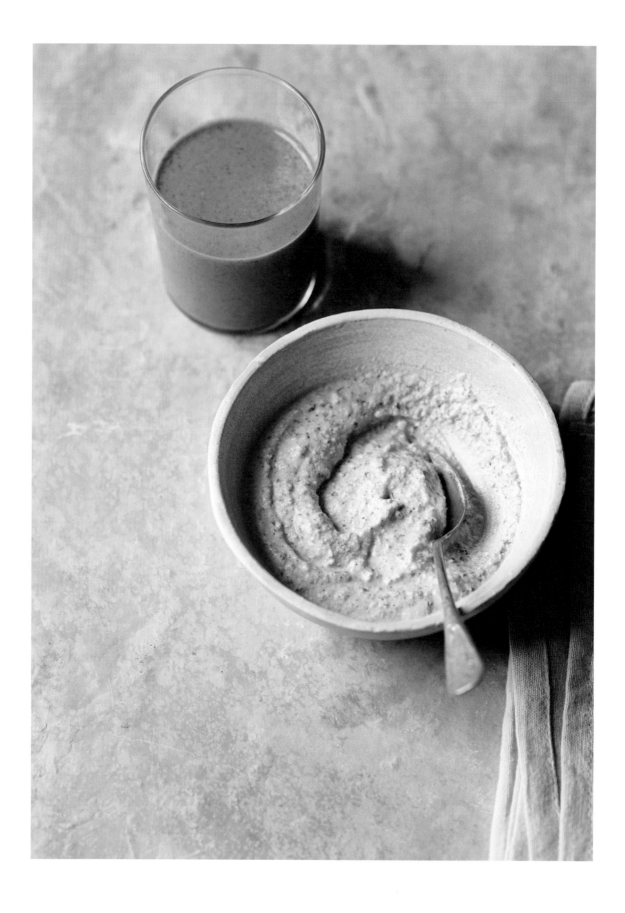

the immunity smoothie

Packed with vitamins A, C and E, which are fundamental in supporting our immune system, this antioxidant-rich smoothie is also a great source of magnesium. It contains protein and fats, and is an excellent way to consume a nutrient-dense 'meal' when you may not feel up to eating. I use coconut water in this smoothie as it is a good source of important minerals such as magnesium, manganese and potassium.

Serves 1

large handful of spinach

3 Tbsp cantaloupe melon

2 Tbsp almond nut butter

2 Tbsp flax seeds (linseeds)

1 kiwi fruit, peeled

handful of ice, plus extra to serve (optional)

200ml (7fl oz/scant 1 cup) water or coconut water

df   gf   vg

1 / Place all the ingredients except the water/coconut water into a blender. Add half of the water and blend for 1 minute on high power. Add the remainder of the water and blend until smooth.

2 / Serve immediately, adding extra ice, if desired.

options
Use coconut oil in place of the nut butter if you have a nut allergy.

tips
You can use any fruit, seeds or nut butter you have to hand – experiment!

banana and almond breakfast pot

Almonds are rich in nutrients such as fibre and healthy fats, and are an excellent source of vitamin E, which protects your cells from damage. Bananas are another good source of fibre, and also potassium, vitamin B6, vitamin C and other antioxidants and phytonutrients. A high proportion of starch in unripe bananas is resistant starch, which passes through your gut undigested. Then, in your large intestine, this starch is fermented by bacteria to form butyrate, a short-chain fatty acid, which appears to have beneficial effects on gut health.

Serves 2

200g (7oz/1½ cups) whole almonds

150ml (5fl oz/⅔ cup) dairy, nut or oat milk, or more as needed

1 medium banana, frozen

2 tsp almond nut butter

1 tsp vanilla extract

df   gf   vg

1 / Place the almonds in a bowl, cover them with water, and leave overnight.

2 / The next day, drain the soaked nuts, then place the nuts in a blender with the milk, banana, nut butter and vanilla extract. Blitz until smooth (adding more milk, if required).

3 / Divide the mixture between 2 small bowls and pop in the fridge to chill.

tips
Experiment with different nut butters: peanut butter and hazelnut butter both taste great in this recipe.

Always keep some peeled and chopped bananas in the freezer to add to smoothies.

Make your own Nut or Oat Milk to use in this recipe (see page 201).

raspberry chia bowl

This is a delicious and nutritious plant-based breakfast made from chia seeds, which are a good source of omega-3 fatty acids, fibre, iron and calcium. Cinnamon is loaded with powerful antioxidants, such as polyphenols, and has anti-inflammatory properties. In fact, in a study that compared the antioxidant activity of 26 spices, cinnamon was the clear winner – even beating 'superfoods' such as garlic.

Serves 2

4 Tbsp chia seeds

250ml (8fl oz/1 cup) dairy, nut or oat milk

1 tsp ground cinnamon

1 tsp vanilla extract

2 Tbsp frozen raspberries

2 Tbsp ground almonds, to serve

<u>df</u> <u>gf</u> <u>vg</u>

1 / Place all the ingredients except the raspberries into a lidded container and mix well. Then, add the frozen raspberries and mix until combined.

2/ Cover and refrigerate for 2–3 hours, or overnight if possible.

3 / Serve with the ground almonds sprinkled on top.

tips
You can use any fresh or frozen berries for this recipe. I like to make it with frozen mango, which is delicious.

Make your own Nut or Oat Milk to use in this recipe (see page 201).

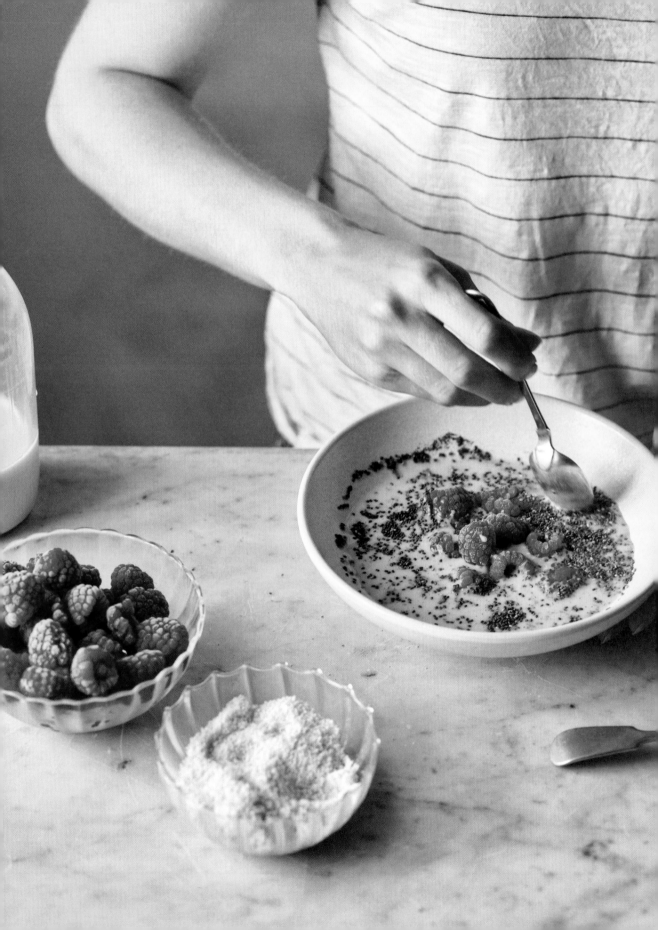

figgy apple and cinnamon porridge

Oats are high in antioxidants and polyphenols, and a great source of the minerals manganese, phosphorus, magnesium, copper, iron and zinc. They are also high in the soluble fibre beta-glucan, which has numerous benefits, including helping to reduce cholesterol and blood-sugar levels, promoting satiety and boosting healthy gut bacteria.

Serves 2

80g (3oz/scant 1 cup) jumbo or rolled oats (oatmeal/old-fashioned oats), gluten-free if necessary

300ml (10fl oz/1¼ cups) dairy, nut or oat milk, or more as needed

2 apples, grated

1 tsp ground cinnamon

1 Tbsp finely sliced dried figs

yoghurt of choice, to serve

df gf vg

1 / Combine the oats and milk in a saucepan and bring to the boil, then reduce the heat and gently simmer for 4–5 minutes, frequently stirring (add more milk, if required).

2/ Stir in the grated apple and cinnamon. Divide between bowls, sprinkle the sliced figs on top, and serve with yoghurt of choice.

tips
This porridge tastes delicious when served with coconut yoghurt.

Make your own Nut or Oat Milk to use in this recipe (see page 201).

no-flour banana pancakes

These no-flour banana pancakes are a brilliant way to start the day, as bananas are nutritional powerhouses, packed with energy-giving carbohydrate and heart-healthy potassium. The pancakes are super-quick to make and children love them, too!

Serves 2 / Makes 4–6

2 large bananas

2 eggs

1 tsp ground cinnamon

1 tsp oil, or more as needed

maple syrup, to serve

df gf

1 / Mash the bananas in a bowl, then add the eggs and cinnamon and stir well.

2 / Gently heat the oil in a frying pan (skillet) over a low heat. Add a spoonful of the batter and cook for 2–3 minutes until set, then flip and cook the other side for the same time. Continue until all the batter has been used up, adding more oil to the pan as necessary.

3 / Serve with maple syrup.

options
For a vegan option, replace the eggs with 1 Tbsp apple sauce and a splash of water.

overnight chocolate oats

Oats are nutrient dense, containing numerous vitamins and minerals as well as being high in powerful antioxidants. I make this breakfast with raw cacao powder, which is one of the best food sources of magnesium – a mineral essential for energy production. Raw cacao powder is also a source of several minerals, including iron, potassium, copper, zinc, manganese and selenium. In addition to this, raw cacao also contains a compound called phenylethylamine (PEA), which is believed to boost energy levels and mood.

Serves 2

50g (2oz/½ cup) jumbo or rolled oats (oatmeal/old-fashioned oats), gluten-free if necessary

250ml (8fl oz/generous 1 cup) organic Greek yoghurt

125ml (4fl oz/½ cup) dairy, nut or oat milk

2–3 Tbsp raw cacao powder or unsweetened cocoa powder

4 tsp maple syrup

gf

1 / Add all the ingredients in the listed order to a container with a tight-fitting lid and stir to combine. Put the lid on firmly and place in the fridge overnight or for at least 8 hours.

2 / Stir before serving.

options
For a vegan or dairy-free option, replace the Greek yoghurt with soy or coconut yoghurt, and use a nut or oat milk.

tips
If you don't have maple syrup you can use honey instead.

Make your own Nut or Oat Milk to use in this recipe (see page 201).

nutty maple granola

Nuts are a good plant-based source of protein, as well being a great source of several micronutrients, including vitamin E, magnesium and selenium. In fact, Brazil nuts are the best source of selenium out there, and selenium plays a very important role in supporting your immune system. It helps reduce inflammation and promotes immunity by lowering oxidative stress in your body. Additionally, studies have shown that while increased blood levels of selenium enhance the immune response, a deficiency may harm immune cells and their function. Selenium also plays a role in the regeneration of vitamins C and E, which help increase your immune system's function. Nuts also contain anti-inflammatory properties and are high in fibre, which helps you to feel full, decreases calorie absorption and improves gut health.

Serves 4

50g (2oz/3½ Tbsp) coconut oil (see Tip)

2–3 Tbsp maple syrup

1 tsp ground cinnamon

1 tsp vanilla or almond extract

1 egg white

50g (2oz/½ cup) rolled oats (oatmeal/old-fashioned oats), gluten-free if necessary

200g (7oz/scant 2 cups) mix of brazil nuts, almonds, hazelnuts and pecans, chopped

4 Tbsp ground flax seed (linseed)

150ml (5fl oz/¾ cup) yoghurt of choice (organic live natural (plain) yoghurt or coconut yoghurt), to serve

df gf

1 / Preheat the oven to 120°C (250°F/gas ½) and grease a baking sheet or line it with baking paper or a silicone baking mat.

2 / In a saucepan over a low heat, gently heat the coconut oil, maple syrup and cinnamon until melted. Remove from the heat, add the vanilla extract, and stir well. Set aside and let cool.

3 / Once the mixture is cool, add the egg white and mix well.

4 / In a bowl, combine the oats, nuts and ground flax seed. Pour in the cooled coconut oil and maple syrup mixture, stirring well.

5 / Spread the mixture over the baking sheet, separating it into small mounds. Bake in the oven for 1–1½ hours until golden, turning the mixture 2–3 times during the cooking time.

6 / Allow to cool and serve with yoghurt.

options
For a vegan option, replace the egg white with either 1 Tbsp apple sauce, ½ mashed banana or 1 Tbsp chickpea (gram) flour.

tips
You can use any combination of nuts and seeds – try experimenting.

If you don't have maple syrup to hand, you can use honey instead.

Make your own Coconut Oil to use in this recipe (see page 200).

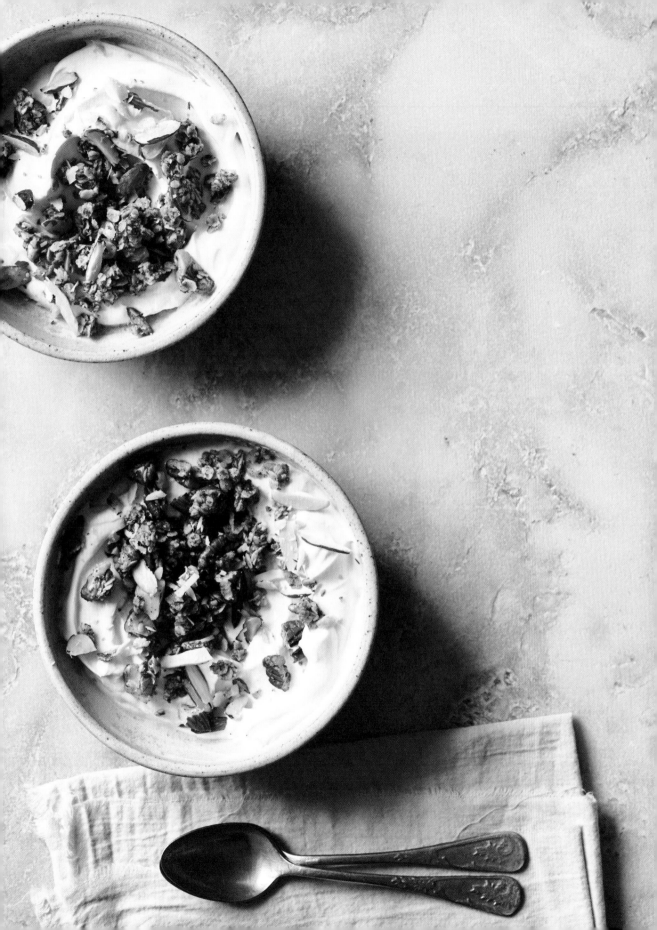

portobello mushrooms with kale and feta

Portobello mushrooms are mature, white button mushrooms and a healthy, edible type of fungus. They are a great source of the B vitamins, antioxidants and phytonutrients, such as CLA and L-ergothioneine, selenium, copper, potassium and phosphorus. I love using kale in this dish as, out of all the super-healthy greens, kale is king. It is one of the most nutrient-dense foods available and contains more vitamin C than an orange. Kale also contains several potent antioxidants, including quercetin and kaempferol, which have numerous health benefits.

Serves 2

2 Tbsp olive oil

120g (4½oz/3 cups) chopped kale, tough stems removed

50g (2oz) feta, crumbled

4 large portobello mushrooms, stalks removed

small handful of fresh thyme, chopped

gf

1 / Preheat the oven to 200°C (400°F/gas 6).

2 / Gently heat 1 tablespoon of the olive oil in a large pan over a low–medium heat. Add the kale and sauté for 5 minutes, then add the feta and cook for a further 1–2 minutes.

3 / Meanwhile, place the mushrooms on a baking sheet with the gills facing up, brush with the remaining olive oil and top with the kale and feta mixture. Pop in the oven and cook for 15 minutes.

4 / Serve sprinkled with the thyme.

options
For a vegan or dairy-free option, omit the feta and replace with nutritional yeast.

tips
You can substitute the portobello mushrooms for red (bell) peppers or even aubergine (eggplant).

If you don't have fresh thyme, use 1 tsp of dried thyme or dried oregano.

poached egg and mushroom hash

Eggs are among the most nutritious foods on the planet, so I love to eat them for breakfast and brunch, especially in this hash. Mushrooms contain B vitamins as well as the potent antioxidant selenium, which helps support the immune system and prevent damage to cells and tissues. In particular, button mushrooms are one of the few non-animal sources of vitamin D.

Serves 2

1 Tbsp olive oil

1 red onion, sliced

250g (9oz/3¾ cups) button mushrooms, sliced

small handful of fresh thyme

250g (9oz/1½ cups) fresh tomatoes, chopped

1 tsp paprika

1 tsp sunflower seeds

2 tsp cider vinegar or white wine vinegar

2 large eggs

freshly ground black pepper

df gf

1 / Gently heat the oil in a large frying pan (skillet) with a lid over a low–medium heat. Add the onion and cook for about 5 minutes until softened. Add the mushrooms and thyme and cook, stirring frequently, for 5 minutes, or until the mushrooms are tender. Reduce the heat to low and add the tomatoes and paprika. Cover the pan with the lid and cook for 5 minutes, adding the sunflower seeds in the last minute of cooking.

2 / Meanwhile, bring a saucepan of water to the boil, add the vinegar, then reduce the heat to low and crack the eggs into the water. Poach for 4–5 minutes.

3 / To serve, top the mushroom hash with the poached eggs and season with freshly ground black pepper.

options
For a vegan option, replace the eggs with smoked tofu.

tips
If you don't have fresh tomatoes, use a can of chopped tomatoes.

If you don't have any fresh thyme, use 1 tsp dried thyme or dried mixed herbs.

Also, experiment with different seeds, such as sunflower, pumpkin or flax seeds (linseeds).

poached eggs with spinach and walnuts

Spinach is thought to be of Persian origin, and by the 12th century had been introduced to Europe, where it became synonymous with good health. It is well known for its nutritional qualities and is rich in iron, which plays a central role in the function of red blood cells and also helps to transport oxygen around the body. Spinach is also an excellent source of vitamins K, A and C, and folate, as well as being a good source of manganese, magnesium, iron and vitamin B2.

Serves 2

2 tsp cider vinegar or white wine vinegar

4 medium or large eggs

2 tsp olive oil

350g (12oz/7 cups) spinach, chopped

pinch of paprika

2 tsp chopped walnuts

freshly ground black pepper

df gf

1 / Bring a large saucepan of water to the boil, add the vinegar, then reduce the heat to low and crack the eggs into the water. Poach for 4–5 minutes.

2 / Meanwhile, heat the oil in a large pan over a low–medium heat. Add the spinach, sprinkle with paprika, and allow to wilt for 2 minutes.

3 / Drain the spinach of any excess liquid in a sieve (strainer), then arrange on plates and top with the poached eggs. Season with freshly ground black pepper and sprinkle over the chopped walnuts.

options
For a vegan option, replace the eggs with 150g (5½oz) smoked tofu.

tips
You can use any nuts you have to hand – toasted pine nuts work really well in this dish.

If you fancy a spicier dish, spice it up by adding ½ tsp ground turmeric and ½ tsp ground cumin.

turmeric scramble

Tofu is a good plant-based protein source, which contains all nine essential amino acids. It is also a valuable source of iron, calcium, manganese and phosphorus. In addition, it contains magnesium, zinc, copper and vitamin B1. I use turmeric a lot in my recipes, as it is a potent anti-inflammatory and antioxidant – its most active compound, curcumin, has many evidence-based health benefits.

Serves 2

2 tsp olive oil

200g (7oz) firm tofu, chopped

1 garlic clove, finely chopped

1 tsp ground turmeric

large handful of spinach, chopped

freshly ground black pepper

2 slices wholegrain or gluten-free bread, toasted, to serve

df gf vg

1 / Heat the oil in a frying pan (skillet) over a low–medium heat. Add the tofu and garlic and gently fry for 5 minutes, then remove to a plate and set aside.

2 / Add the turmeric and spinach to the pan, along with a twist of black pepper, and cook for 2–3 minutes, adding a splash of water, if required, until the spinach has wilted. Return the tofu mixture to the pan and cook, stirring continuously, for 5–8 minutes until the scramble is the desired consistency.

3 / Season with freshly ground black pepper, and serve with a slice of toasted wholegrain bread.

tips
Black pepper significantly enhances the benefits of the turmeric, so make sure you add a generous twist of freshly ground black pepper.

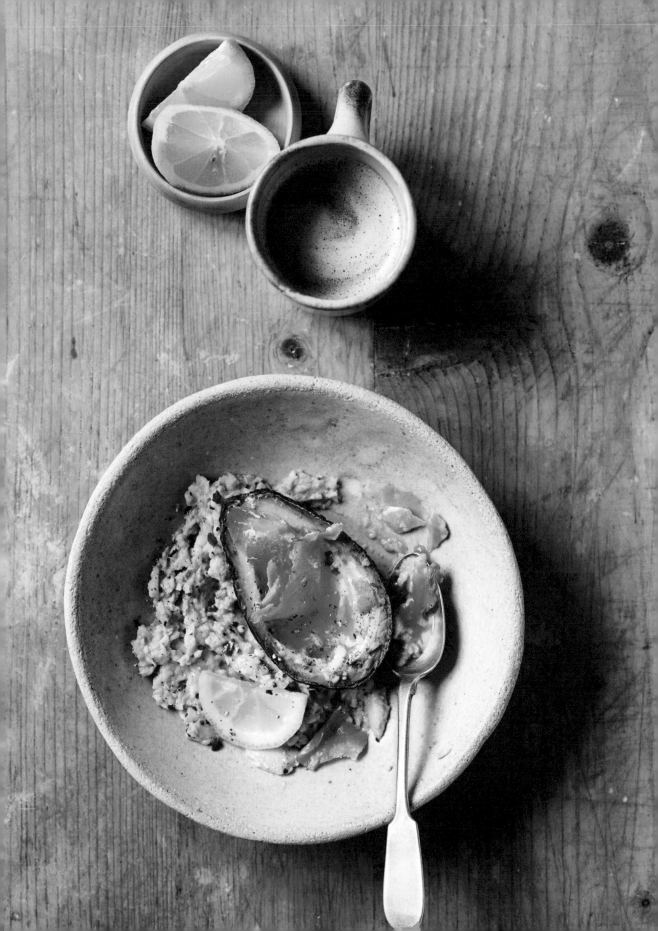

baked eggs in avocado

This has to be my favourite breakfast dish, as it combines two of the most nutritious foods out there – eggs and avocado! Eggs are an excellent source of high-quality yet inexpensive protein, and more than half the protein found in an egg is in the egg white, which also includes vitamin B2. In addition, eggs are also good sources of immunity-supporting vitamin D, vitamins B6 and B12, and minerals such as selenium, iron, zinc and copper. Avocados are an excellent source of monounsaturated fat and fibre – in fact, they have more soluble fibre than any other fruit. They are also a good source of B vitamins and vitamins C, E and K, and the minerals potassium, copper and iron. In addition to containing all these important nutrients, avocados also provide the powerful antioxidants beta-carotene and lutein, as well as omega-3 fatty acids.

Serves 2

1 large avocado

2 medium or large eggs

pinch of paprika

3 slices smoked salmon, thinly sliced

¼ tsp chilli (red pepper) flakes

squeeze of lemon juice

freshly ground black pepper

1 / Preheat the oven to 200°C (400°F/gas 6).

2 / Halve and de-stone the avocado. Use a spoon to scoop out the flesh from each half into a mixing bowl, ensuring you leave a 1.5cm (½in) depth of avocado flesh still attached to the skins. Place the avocado halves in a baking tin (pan), crack one egg into each half and sprinkle with paprika. Place the thinly sliced smoked salmon on top, then pop into the oven to bake for 8–10 minutes.

3 / Meanwhile, mash the avocado flesh in the bowl, then add the chilli flakes and lemon juice and mix well.

4 / Remove the baked avocado halves from the oven, season with freshly ground black pepper, and serve with the mashed avocado on the side.

options
For a vegan option, replace the eggs with chopped walnuts – avocado and walnuts are a winning combination. If you replace the eggs with walnuts, make sure you reduce the cooking time to 5–7 minutes.

miso soup

Miso means 'fermented beans' in Japanese, and in Japan it is traditional to eat miso soup once a day, even at breakfast. It is believed to stimulate digestion and energize the body. Miso paste is made from fermented soybeans and grains and contains millions of beneficial bacteria. In addition, miso is a complete source of protein and rich in a variety of nutrients and beneficial plant compounds.

Serves 4

3–4 tsp instant dashi (Japanese stock) or 3 tsp vegetable bouillon powder

4 spring onions (scallions), finely sliced

2 Tbsp miso paste

200g (7oz) silken tofu, cubed

1 Tbsp sweet rice wine

1 Tbsp soy sauce

df vg

1 / Bring 800ml (27fl oz/scant 3½ cups) water to the boil in a saucepan and stir in the dashi or vegetable bouillon powder. Add the sliced onions and simmer for 2 minutes.

2 / Meanwhile, put the miso paste into a small bowl, add a ladleful of the hot broth and whisk until smooth. Add the paste to the saucepan and whisk to combine. Add the tofu, sweet rice wine and soy sauce and gently heat through without boiling.

3 / Serve immediately.

options
For a gluten-free option, replace the soy sauce with tamari.

tips
Try adding wakame seaweed to the recipe. It has a subtly sweet flavour that counterbalances the umami taste of the miso and dashi. Also, the chewiness adds bulk to the soup, as well as providing a contrasting texture.

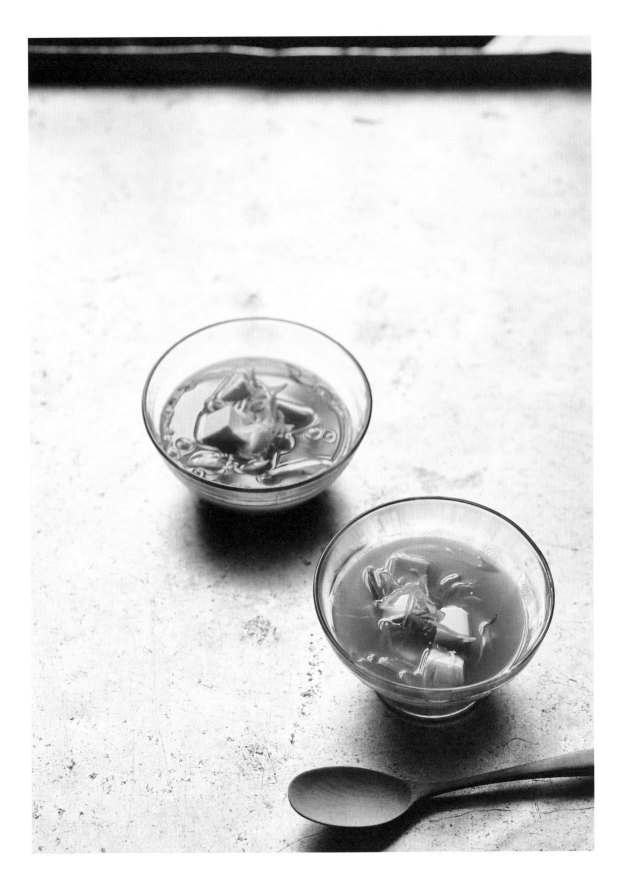

chicken and vegetable soup

Chicken is high in protein, which helps support the immune system, and is also a good source of vitamins and minerals, such as B vitamins, which support immunity and aid digestion. It is also high in tryptophan, which helps your body produce serotonin, resulting in enhanced mood. This soup is loaded with antioxidant-rich vegetables and the ginger not only gives it a kick, but is among the healthiest spices on the planet – it is packed with bioactive compounds that have powerful benefits for your brain and body.

Serves 4

2 Tbsp olive oil

1 onion, finely chopped

1 garlic clove, finely chopped

3cm (1in) piece of fresh root ginger, grated

2 skinless and boneless chicken thighs, cubed

3 carrots, sliced

1 medium sweet potato, roughly chopped

1 head broccoli, roughly chopped

freshly ground black pepper

df gf

1 / Heat the oil in a saucepan over a medium heat. Add the onion, garlic and ginger and cook until lightly browned. Add the chicken, carrots, sweet potato and broccoli, along with 850ml (29fl oz/3½ cups) water, and simmer over a low heat for about 1 hour (if it starts to look dry, you can add another 3 tablespoons of water during cooking).

2 / Remove from the heat and transfer to a food processor or blender and blitz until creamy and smooth. Season to taste with freshly ground black pepper

options
For a vegan option, replace the chicken with 1 x 400g (14oz) can drained chickpeas (garbanzo beans).

tips
This is a really versatile recipe – you can use whatever vegetables you have to hand. Pumpkin, celery and leeks all work well here.

pea, basil and mint soup

This is a very quick and nutritious soup. Green peas are a good source of plant-based protein, and contain several different vitamins and minerals, as well as being high in fibre. The basil not only makes this soup taste delicious, but it also provides beneficial plant compounds that have antioxidant, anti-inflammatory and other health properties.

Serves 4

1 Tbsp olive oil

1 white onion, finely chopped

500g (1lb 2oz/4 cups) frozen petits pois

small handful of basil leaves, chopped

small handful of mint leaves, chopped

1 tsp sea salt (kosher salt)

freshly ground black pepper

df gf vg

1 / Gently heat the oil in a saucepan over a medium heat. Add the onion and cook for about 5 minutes, or until softened. Add two-thirds of the peas along with 600ml (20fl oz/2½ cups) water and half each of the basil and mint. Stir in the salt and bring to the boil, then reduce the heat and simmer for 20 minutes, or until the peas are tender.

2 / Remove from the heat and transfer the soup to a food processor or blender along with the remaining peas, basil and mint (you may need to do this in batches). Blitz until creamy and smooth.

3 / Transfer back to the saucepan and gently heat through.

4 / Season with freshly ground black pepper and serve.

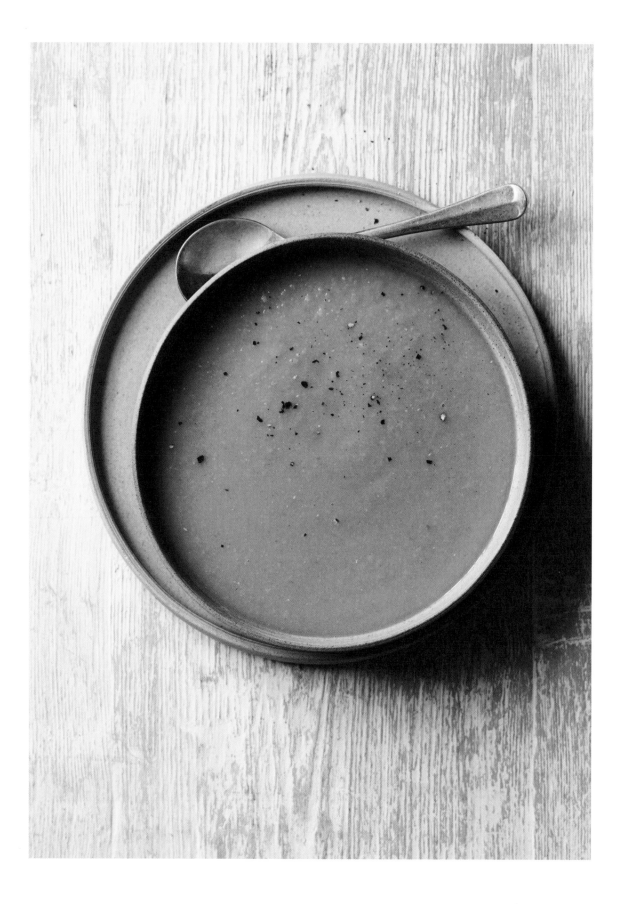

lentil and butternut squash soup

Lentils are an inexpensive plant-based protein source loaded with B vitamins, magnesium, zinc and potassium. As they are made up of over 25 per cent protein, they're an excellent meat alternative. They're also a valuable source of iron, a mineral that is sometimes lacking in a plant-based diet. In addition, they're fibre-rich, which is exactly what we need to help support gut function and overall gut health.

Serves 4

2 Tbsp olive oil

2 red onions, finely chopped

2 garlic cloves, finely chopped

1 medium butternut squash, peeled and roughly chopped

110g (4oz/⅔ cup) dried red lentils

1 litre (34fl oz/generous 4 cups) hot vegetable stock (bouillon)

juice of ½ lemon

freshly ground black pepper

1 / Gently heat the oil in a saucepan over a medium heat. Add the onions and garlic and cook for about 5 minutes until softened. Add the butternut squash, lentils and hot stock and stir well. Reduce the heat to low and simmer for 30–35 minutes until the butternut squash is soft and the lentils are cooked.

2 / Remove from the heat and transfer the soup to a food processor or blender. Add the lemon juice and blitz until creamy and smooth. Season to taste with freshly ground black pepper.

tips

You can use any kind of dried lentils you have to hand – red, yellow, brown, green or black. I tend to use red or yellow lentils for this soup, as they provide a sweet, nutty flavour and a lovely colour when combined with the butternut squash. Also, if you don't have dried lentils, you can always use canned.

Substitute pumpkin for the butternut squash, if you prefer.

This tastes super with a little 'heat', so try spicing it up with 1 tsp chilli powder or ground cumin.

roasted pepper and tomato soup

Red peppers are very high in vitamin C, and also include good amounts of vitamins K, E and A, folate and potassium. They also contain antioxidants such as capsanthin (responsible for giving them their brilliant colour), violaxanthin, lutein, quercetin and luteolin, which are all associated with many health benefits.

Serves 4

3 red (bell) peppers, deseeded and halved

1 red onion, halved

500g (1lb 2 oz) ripe tomatoes, halved

3 garlic cloves, peeled and left whole

3 Tbsp olive oil

2 celery sticks, chopped

900ml (30fl oz/scant 4 cups) hot vegetable stock (bouillon), or more as needed

2 Tbsp tomato purée (paste)

1 Tbsp sundried tomato paste

freshly ground black pepper

1 Tbsp chopped fresh basil, to garnish

df gf vg

1 / Preheat the oven to 200°C (400°F/gas 6).

2 / Arrange the peppers, onion, tomatoes and garlic on a baking sheet. Drizzle with 2 tablespoons of the olive oil, then roast on the top shelf of the oven for 30–35 minutes until tender.

3 / Meanwhile, heat the remaining tablespoon of olive oil in a saucepan with a lid over a low–medium heat and gently sauté the celery for 3–4 minutes. Add the hot stock, tomato purée and sundried tomato paste and bring to the boil, then reduce the heat, cover and simmer for 8–10 minutes.

4 / Meanwhile, gently remove the outer skin from the roasted peppers and tomatoes. Roughly chop them. Chop the onion and garlic, then add to the saucepan along with the peppers and tomatoes. Cook for 5–6 minutes over a low–medium heat, stirring frequently.

5 / Remove from the heat, transfer the soup to a food processor or blender and blitz until creamy and smooth (add a little more stock, if required, to reach the desired consistency). Season to taste with freshly ground black pepper.

6 / Serve, sprinkled with the fresh basil.

tips
In place of fresh tomatoes, you can use canned chopped tomatoes, and if you don't have fresh basil to hand, you can use dried basil instead.

Spice this up by adding 1 tsp chilli powder or ground cumin.

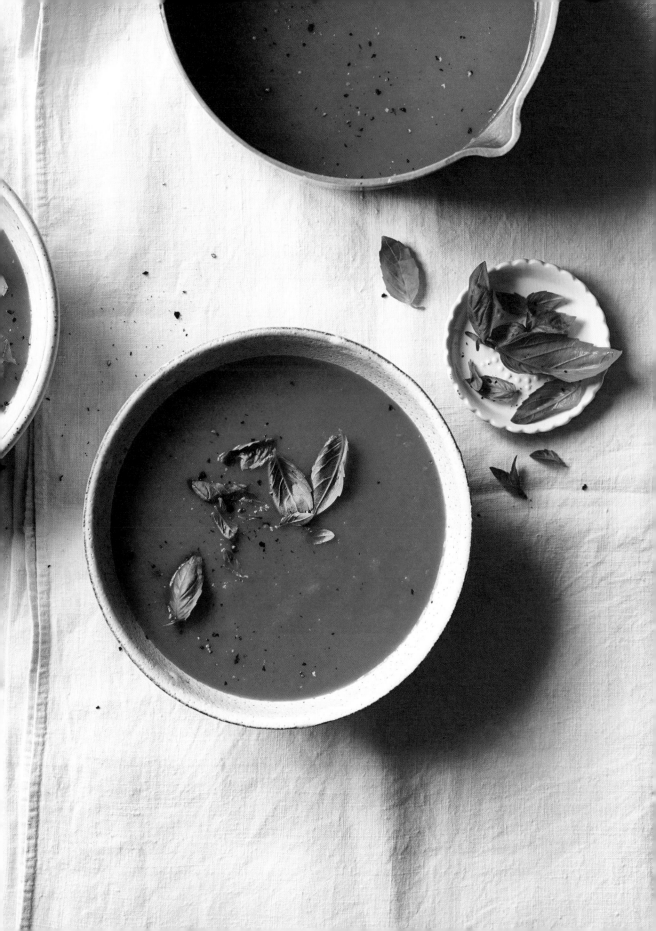

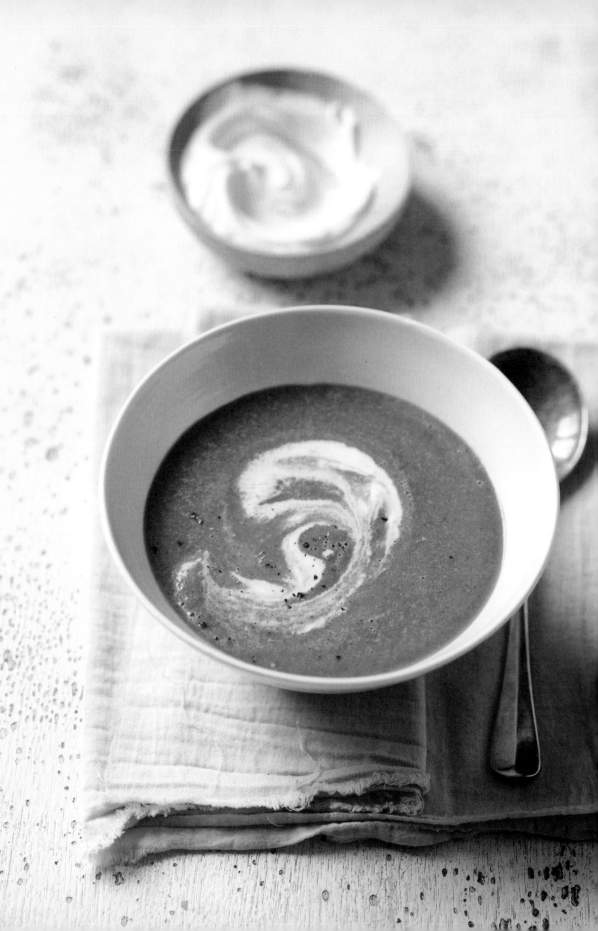

spinach and watercress soup

Watercress is part of the Brassicaceae family of vegetables, which also includes cauliflower, cabbage and kale. It is a good source of vitamin C, which supports immunity, and is also an excellent source of vitamin K, which is a fat-soluble vitamin necessary for blood clotting and healthy bones. Watercress also contains lutein and zeaxanthin, which are antioxidant compounds in the carotenoid family and very beneficial to our health.

Serves 4

1 Tbsp olive oil

1 white onion, finely chopped

1 garlic clove, finely chopped

150g (5½oz/3 cups) watercress, chopped

150g (5½oz/3 cups) spinach, chopped

700ml (24fl oz/3 cups) freshly boiled water

freshly ground black pepper

4 Tbsp crème fraîche, to serve (optional)

df gf vg

1 / Heat the oil in a saucepan over a low–medium heat. Add the onion and garlic and cook for about 5 minutes, or until softened. Add the watercress and cook for 1 minute, then add the spinach and cook for a further minute. Add the boiling water, stir, and cook for a further 2 minutes.

2 / Remove from the heat, transfer the soup to a food processor or blender, and blitz until creamy and smooth. Season to taste with freshly ground black pepper.

3 / Serve with a drizzle of crème fraîche, if using.

tips
In place of crème fraîche you can use coconut yoghurt.

summertime avocado and cucumber soup

I've already mentioned on page 79 how wonderful avocados are, being my number one go-to food source of monounsaturated fat and containing potent antioxidants. Cucumbers can help lower inflammatory response in the body, and they also contain polyphenols called lignans, which can potentially reduce the risk of cardiovascular disease and certain cancers.

Serves 4

4 small ripe avocados, halved, stone removed and flesh scooped out, plus extra to garnish if desired

4 small cucumbers, peeled and quartered, plus extra to garnish if desired

2 white onions, quartered

2 garlic cloves, peeled

large handful of fresh coriander (cilantro) leaves

juice of ½ lemon

pinch of ground cumin

freshly ground black pepper

df gf vg

1 / Place all the ingredients, except the black pepper, in a food processor or blender. Add 300ml (10fl oz/1¼ cups) water and blitz until smooth and creamy (add a little more water, if required, to reach the desired consistency).

2 / Transfer to the fridge to chill for 50 minutes.

3 / Serve chilled, seasoned with freshly ground black pepper and extra chopped avocado and cucumber if desired.

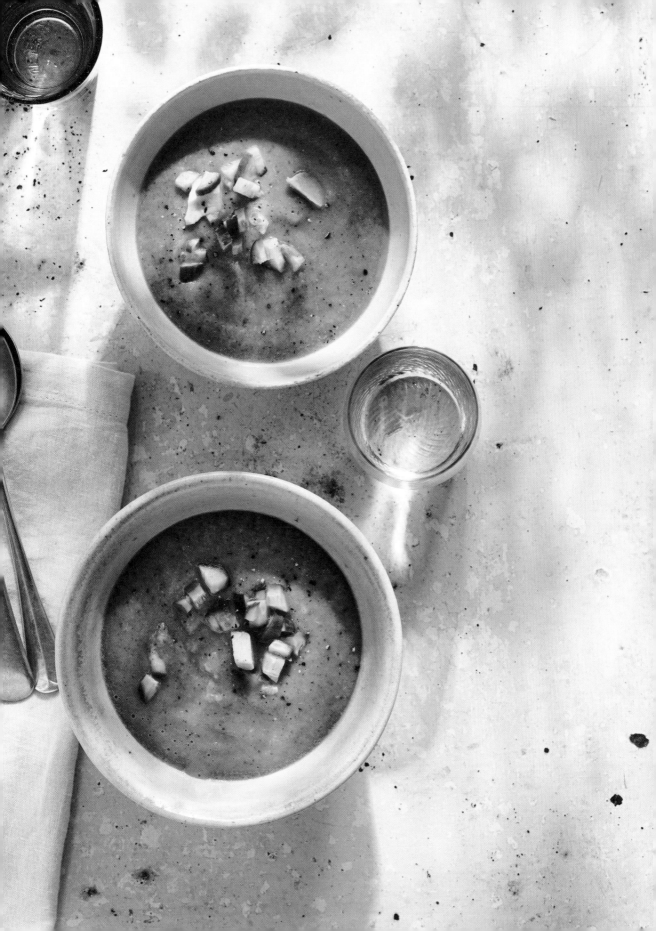

chicken, broccoli and beetroot salad

Packed with essential nutrients, beetroots are a great source of folate, manganese, potassium, iron, vitamin C and fibre. Beetroot (beets) have been associated with numerous health benefits, including improved blood flow, lower blood pressure and increased exercise performance. Many of these benefits are due to their high content of inorganic nitrates. In addition, both beetroot and broccoli contain betaine, which boosts production of the happy hormone, serotonin.

Serves 4

250g (9oz) thin-stemmed broccoli

2 Tbsp olive oil

4 skinless chicken breasts

120g (4½oz/generous 2 cups) watercress

3 spring onions (scallions), finely sliced

juice of ½ lime, plus extra wedges to serve

2 beetroot (beets), peeled and grated

1 tsp nigella (charnushka) seeds

df gf

1 / Bring a large saucepan of water to the boil, then reduce to a simmer and add the broccoli. Cook for 2 minutes, then drain and set aside.

2 / Meanwhile, gently heat 1 tablespoon of the oil in a large sauté pan over a low heat. Add the broccoli and cook for 3 minutes, turning frequently. Set aside on a separate plate.

3 / Brush the chicken breasts with the remaining olive oil, then add to the sauté pan, increase the heat to medium and cook for 5–7 minutes on each side, or until cooked through. Set aside and leave to cool.

4 / Once cool, slice the chicken breasts. Place the watercress in a large bowl and toss through the broccoli, spring onions and lime juice. Add the grated beetroot and sliced chicken, then season with ground black pepper and sprinkle with the nigella seeds.

options
For a vegan option, replace the chicken breasts with chickpeas (garbanzo beans).

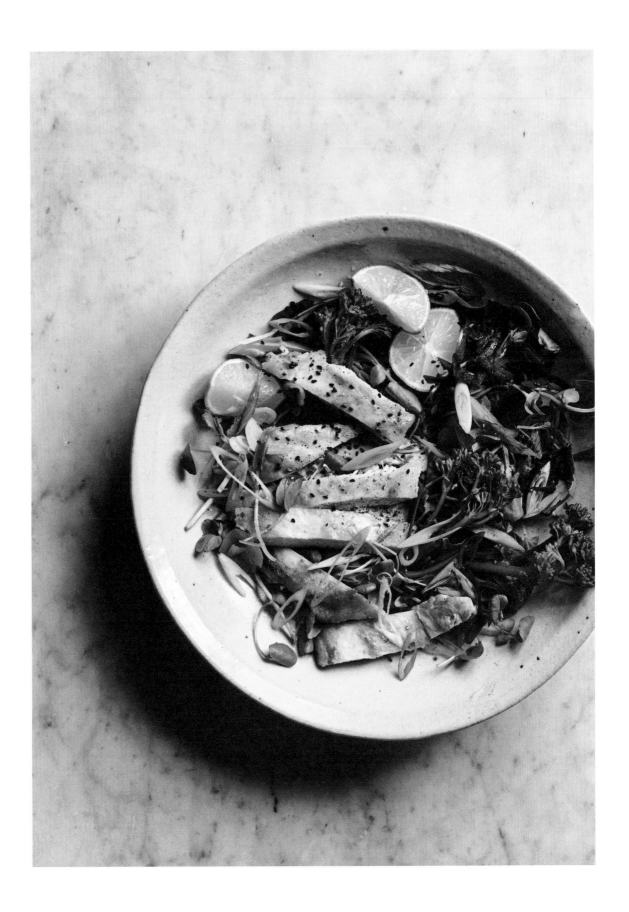

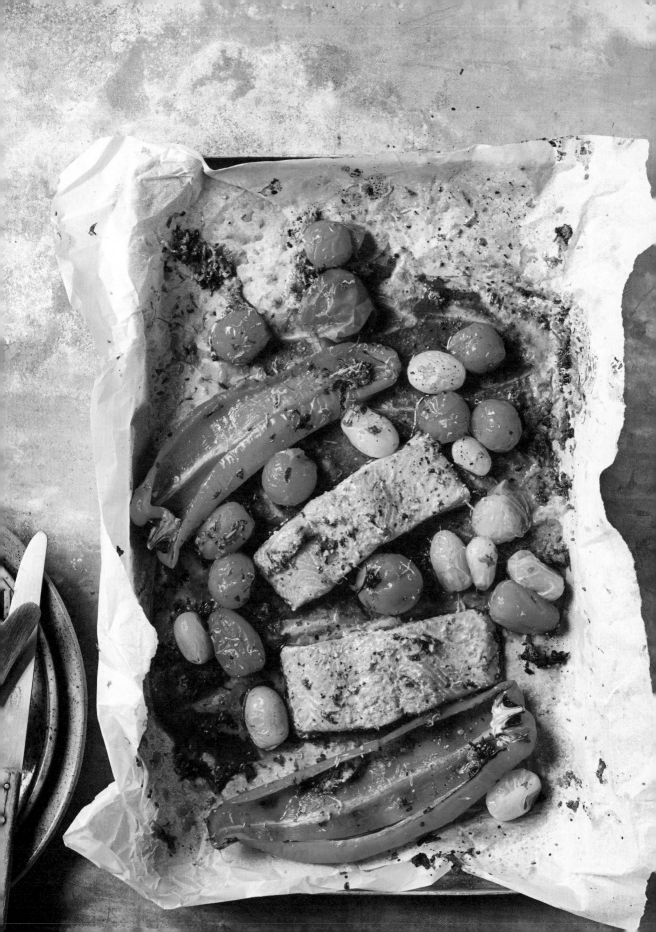

zingy teriyaki salmon salad

Salmon is a fatty fish loaded with healthy omega-3 fatty acids and vitamin D, which plays an extremely important role in supporting our immune systems. However, not all salmon is created equal – farmed salmon contains up to three times more saturated fat than wild salmon. Additionally, wild salmon is higher in vitamin D, and minerals such as iron, zinc and potassium, so do opt for wild salmon over farmed salmon, if possible.

Serves 2

1 Tbsp extra-virgin olive oil

3 tsp soy sauce

zest and juice of 1 lime

2cm (¾in) piece of fresh root ginger, grated

small handful of fresh coriander (cilantro), finely chopped

2 wild salmon fillets

1 red (bell) pepper, halved and deseeded

10 cherry and/or baby heritage tomatoes

salad leaves of your choice, to serve

df

1 / Preheat the oven to 200°C (400°F/gas 6) and line a baking sheet with baking paper or foil.

2 / In a large bowl, mix together the oil, soy sauce, lime zest and juice, ginger and fresh coriander. Place the salmon in the marinade and set aside for 15 minutes.

3 / Place the marinated salmon, pepper halves and tomatoes on the lined baking sheet and cook in the oven for 15 minutes.

4 / Remove and serve on a bed of salad leaves.

options
For a vegan option, replace the salmon with firm tofu, cut into chunks.

For a gluten-free option, replace the soy sauce with tamari.

tips
If you don't have fresh coriander (cilantro) to hand, use 1 tsp ground coriander instead.

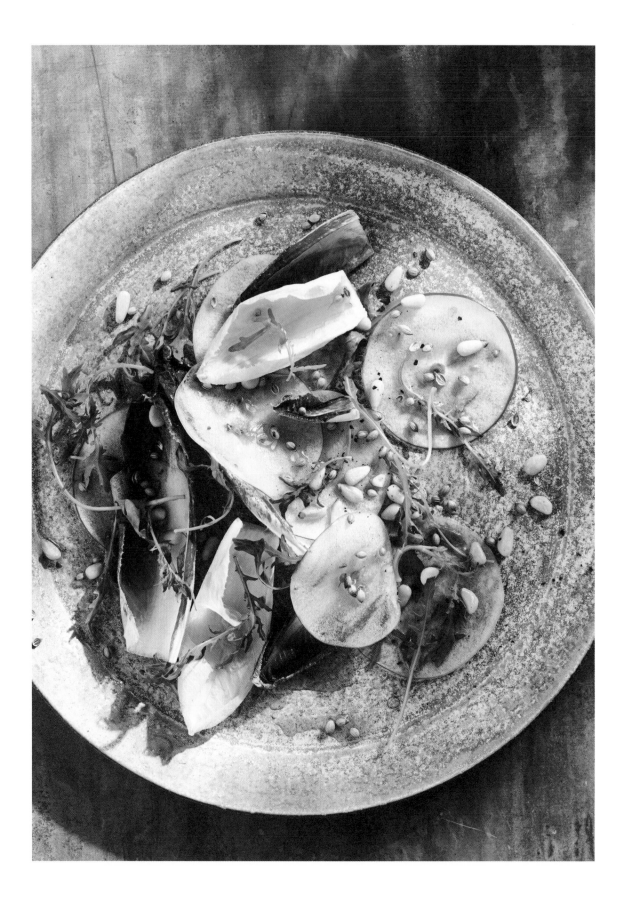

chicory and apple salad

Chicory, also known as endive, is a wonderful vegetable that can be eaten raw or cooked and comes in red and white varieties. I use both in this salad, where the bitter chicory leaves are balanced perfectly by the sweetness of the apple.

Serves 4

2 sweet apples, cored and cut into thin slices

juice of 1 lemon

1–2 tsp olive oil

½ tsp coriander seeds, crushed

2 heads red chicory (endive), leaves separated

2 heads white chicory (endive), leaves separated

120g (4½oz/generous 2 cups) rocket (arugula)

80g (3oz/generous ½ cup) pine nuts

df gf vg

1 / Place the thinly sliced apples in a dish, dress with the lemon juice and olive oil and sprinkle over the coriander seeds.

2 / In a separate dish, toss the chicory leaves together with the rocket. Add the apple slices and juices to the salad leaves, sprinkle with the pine nuts and serve.

tips
You can replace the rocket with watercress or baby spinach.

Be sure to use sweet apples for this salad, the sweeter the better! I use either Fuji or Gala, and they work perfectly with the chicory leaves.

warm chicken and asparagus salad

Chicken is high in protein and lower in fat compared to other animal sources like beef, particularly the breast meat. In addition, chicken is a great source of iron, zinc, selenium and B vitamins. Asparagus is another great source of nutrients, including fibre, folate and vitamins A, K and C.

Serves 4

8 new potatoes, halved if big

1 Tbsp olive oil

3 chicken breasts, sliced

2 garlic cloves, crushed

150g (5½oz) asparagus

2 little gem lettuces, leaves separated

Homemade Vinaigrette (see page 198), to serve

df gf

1 / Bring a large pan of water to the boil, add the potatoes and cook for 10 minutes. Drain and set aside.

2 / Gently heat the olive oil in a sauté pan over a medium heat, add the sliced chicken and cook until golden on all sides. Add the garlic and asparagus and sauté until the chicken is cooked through and the asparagus is lightly browned and tender.

3 / Arrange the lettuce leaves in a large serving dish and top with the chicken, asparagus and potatoes. Drizzle with vinaigrette and serve.

options
For a vegan option, replace the chicken with 300g (10½oz/2 cups) chickpeas (garbanzo beans).

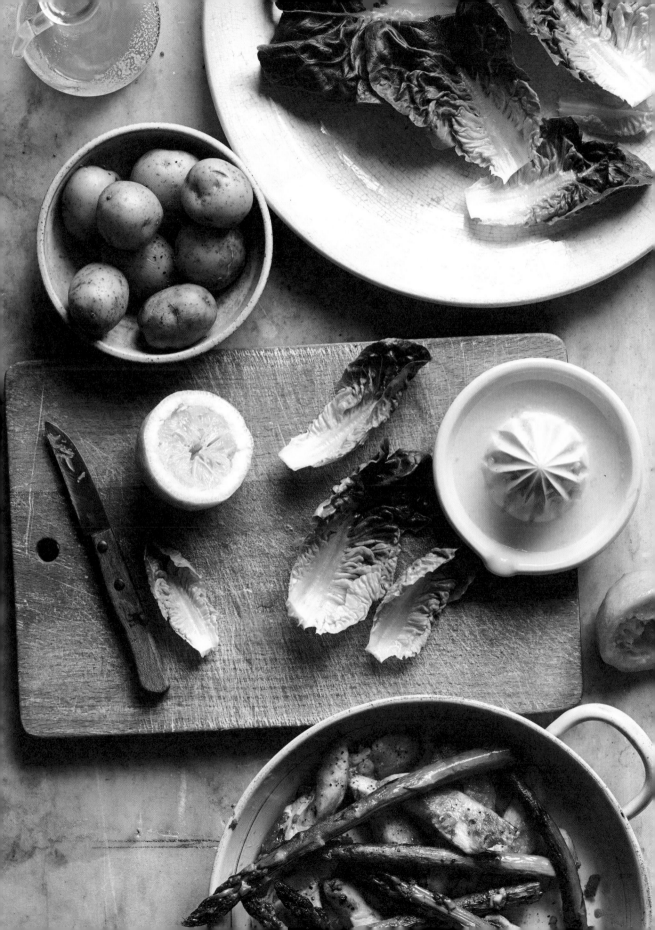

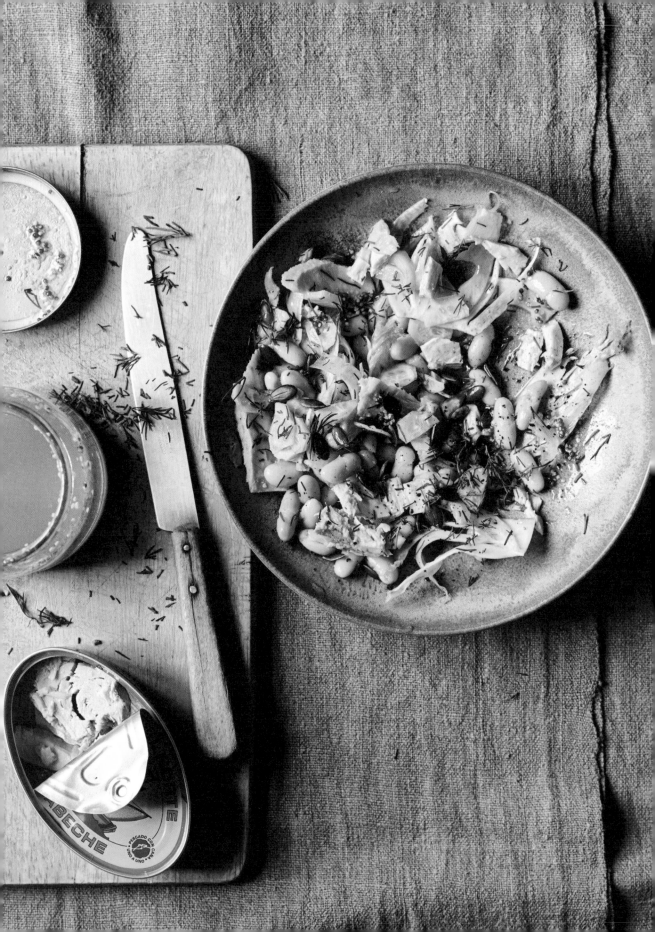

tuna, fennel and bean salad

Tuna in spring water is a super source of protein, and also a good source of phosphorous, iron, magnesium, vitamin A and the B vitamins, niacin and riboflavin. In addition, it has a high content of omega-3 fatty acids, which support the immune, endocrine and cardiovascular systems. The fennel – a great prebiotic food source – works really well with the tuna and beans in this recipe, and it also provides important nutrients such as vitamin C, magnesium, calcium, potassium and manganese. In addition, the powerful antioxidants in fennel, such as quercetin and vitamin C may help to decrease inflammation and levels of inflammatory markers.

Serves 4

zest and juice of 2 lemons

2 tsp wholegrain mustard

2 Tbsp olive oil

2 x 400g (14oz) cans cannellini beans, drained and rinsed

small bunch of dill, chopped

1 small fennel bulb, thinly shaved

1 cucumber, peeled and finely chopped

2 x 150g (5½oz) cans tuna in spring water, drained

2 Tbsp pumpkin seeds

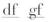

1 / First, make the dressing. Combine the lemon zest and juice, mustard and olive oil in a small container or jar with a tight-fitting lid and shake for 30 seconds.

2 / Meanwhile, put the beans into a large bowl and pour the dressing over, stirring to make sure the beans are evenly coated. Add the dill, fennel and cucumber, then gently stir in the tuna. Sprinkle with the pumpkin seeds and serve.

options
For a vegan option, replace the tuna with extra cannellini beans, or add in some butter (lima) beans.

tips
Tuna does contain mercury, so I would suggest keeping your intake to once a week and opt for a low-sodium variety of canned tuna.

beetroot and carrot salad

Beetroot (beets) are sweet and taste delicious in salads; combined with carrots, they make the perfect combination! Carrots are a particularly good source of beta-carotene, vitamin K, potassium, antioxidants and fibre. They also have a number of health benefits, and have been linked to lower cholesterol levels and improved eye health. This salad tastes delicious with the toasted pine nuts, which pack a nutrient punch, too, being good sources of vitamin E, copper, magnesium and zinc.

Serves 4

4 Tbsp olive oil

juice of ½ lime

3 Tbsp tamari

2 beetroot (beets), peeled and grated

250g (9oz/2 cups) carrots, grated

150g (5½oz/generous 1 cup) pine nuts,

100g (3½oz/¾ cup) sesame seeds

df gf vg

1 / In a bowl, mix together the oil, lime juice and tamari.

2 / In a separate bowl, toss together the grated beetroot and carrots.

3 / Meanwhile, gently toast the pine nuts and sesame seeds in a dry pan over a low heat, frequently turning until lightly browned. Set aside to cool.

4 / Mix the lime and tamari dressing into the grated beetroot and carrot mixture. Once the nuts and seeds are cool, sprinkle them over the salad and serve.

tips
You can use whatever seeds and nuts you have to hand – pumpkin seeds and walnuts also work really well with the beetroot and carrot.

kale and goat's cheese frittata

I love frittatas as they are so quick and straightforward, yet so nutrient dense. This gluten-free vegetarian frittata is packed with kale, which is a cruciferous vegetable like cabbage, broccoli, cauliflower, collard greens and Brussels sprouts. It is super-high in vitamins A, C and K, and antioxidants, such as the flavonoids quercetin and kaempferol. Goat's cheese is also a good source of protein and healthy fats. Additionally, goat's milk contains capric acid, a medium-chain fatty acid that has been shown to possess antibacterial and anti-inflammatory properties.

Serves 4

1 Tbsp olive oil

2 red onions, finely chopped

200g (7oz/5 cups) curly kale, chopped

2 Tbsp balsamic vinegar

8 medium or large eggs, beaten

120g (4½oz) goat's cheese, chopped into chunks

freshly ground black pepper

1 / Preheat the oven to 180°C (350°F/gas 4).

2 / Gently heat the oil in an ovenproof frying pan (skillet) over a low heat. Add the onions and cook for 5 minutes until browned and softened, then add the kale and cook for a further 5–6 minutes. Add the balsamic vinegar and cook for 1 minute. Add the eggs, stir once, then leave to cook over a low–medium heat for 5 minutes until the frittata is turning golden on the bottom and the egg is almost set.

3 / Sprinkle the goat's cheese over the frittata, then transfer the pan to the oven for 10–12 minutes until the cheese bubbles and the frittata is cooked in the middle.

4 / Season to taste with freshly ground black pepper.

sundried tomato, feta and basil omelette

Sundried tomatoes are intensely flavoured and are a concentrated source of nutrients. They provide vitamins C and K, and iron, along with lycopene, an antioxidant associated with lower risk of certain cancers.

Serves 2

2 large ripe tomatoes, finely chopped

2 sundried tomatoes, finely chopped

2 Tbsp feta, crumbled

5 basil leaves, finely chopped

2 spring onions (scallions), finely chopped

2 Tbsp olive oil

4 medium or large eggs, beaten

freshly ground black pepper

To serve:
mixed salad

Crunchy Coleslaw (see page 193)

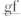

1 / Combine the fresh tomatoes, sundried tomatoes, feta, basil, spring onions and 1 tablespoon of the olive oil in a bowl.

2 / Gently heat the remaining oil in a frying pan (skillet) over a low heat and pour in the eggs. Cook until set and lightly browned, then turn and cook the other side. Tip half of the tomato and feta mixture onto one half of the omelette, fold the other half of the omelette over to enclose the filling, and leave in the pan for a further 45 seconds.

3 / Season to taste with freshly ground black pepper and serve with a mixed salad and some crunchy coleslaw.

options
For a dairy-free option, replace the feta with 1 Tbsp nutritional yeast.

tips
Omelettes are so versatile – you can add anything you have to hand. Try making an omelette filled with finely diced butternut squash, halloumi and chilli – it's one of my absolute favourites. You could also use button mushrooms, smoked salmon and asparagus.

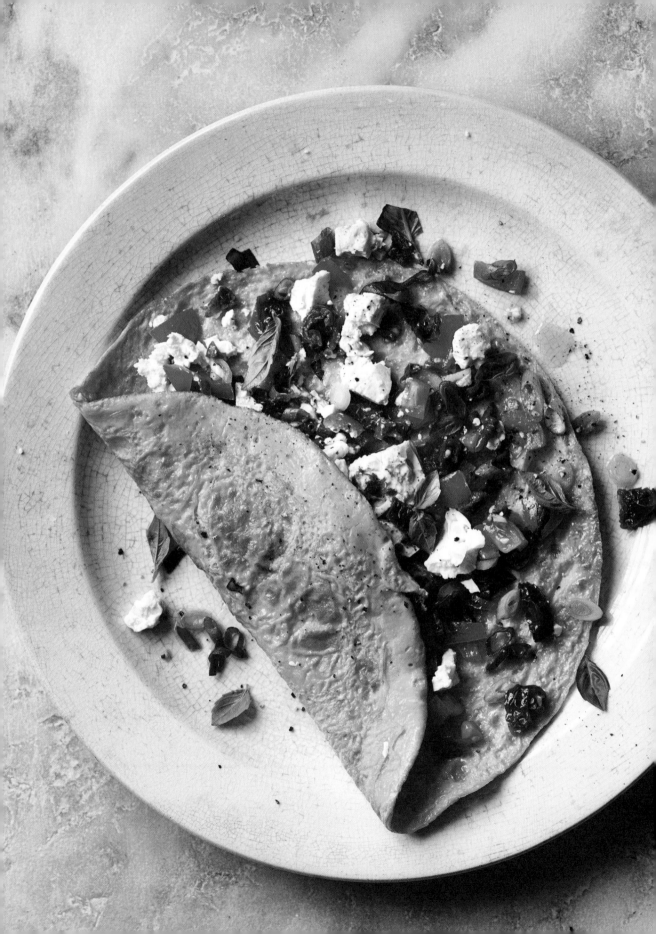

pepper and rocket frittata

I use red bell peppers in this frittata as they are good sources of vitamins K, E and A, folate and potassium. They are also very high in vitamin C and contain powerful antioxidants, such as capsanthin, violaxanthin, lutein, quercetin and luteolin, which have been demonstrated to provide several benefits to health.

Serves 4

1 Tbsp olive oil

2 red (bell) peppers, deseeded and chopped

1 red onion, diced

2 garlic cloves, crushed

4 medium or large eggs

2 handfuls of rocket (arugula), chopped

3 Tbsp pesto

handful of fresh basil, chopped

100g (3½oz) mozzarella, chopped

freshly ground black pepper

gf

1 / Preheat the grill (broiler) to medium-high.

2 / Meanwhile, heat the olive oil in an ovenproof frying pan (skillet) over a low–medium heat. Add the red peppers and cook until softened. Stir in the onion and cook for 3 minutes, then add the crushed garlic and cook for a further 2 minutes.

3 / Meanwhile, whisk the eggs in a bowl along with the rocket, pesto and fresh basil. Season with freshly ground black pepper.

4 / Pour the egg mixture into the frying pan and cook for 3–5 minutes until the bottom of the frittata is almost set. Scatter the mozzarella over the frittata, then pop the pan under the grill for about 10 minutes or until the frittata is cooked in the middle.

tips
Make your own pesto to use in this recipe (see page 199).

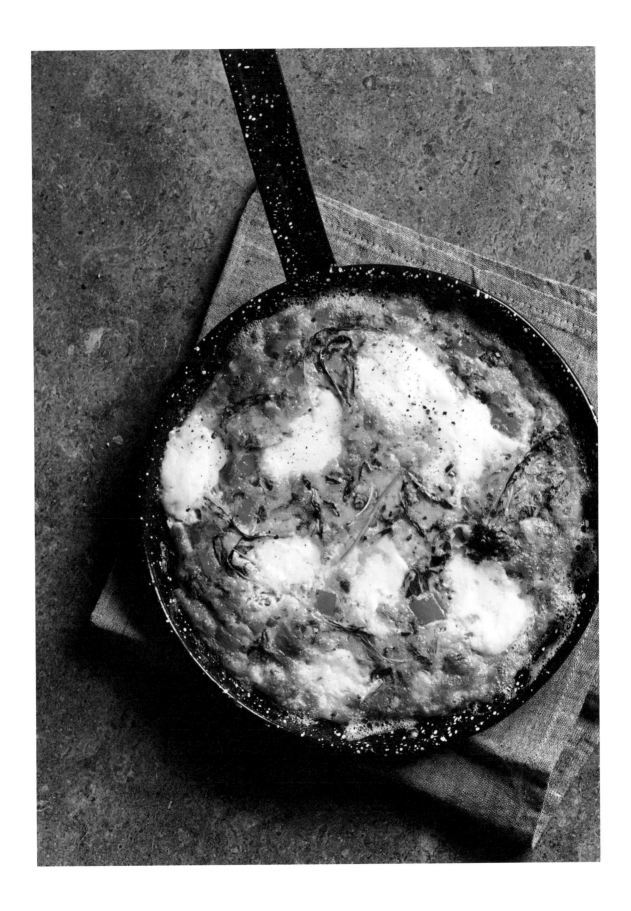

broccoli and potato frittata with a bean salad

Broccoli is a nutritional powerhouse full of vitamins, minerals, fibre and antioxidants. It also contains various bioactive compounds that have been demonstrated to decrease inflammation in your body's tissues. Additionally, eating fibre-rich foods like broccoli may help play a role in maintaining healthy gut function.

Serves 4

120g (4½oz) new potatoes

200g (7oz) Tenderstem broccoli

1 x 400g (14oz) can mixed beans, drained

200g (7oz) green beans, trimmed and halved

2 Tbsp olive oil

2 garlic cloves, crushed

6 medium or large eggs

80g (3oz/⅓ cup) ricotta cheese

1 tsp apple cider vinegar

small bunch of basil, chopped

freshly ground black pepper

1 / Bring a large saucepan of water to the boil and boil the potatoes for 10–12 minutes until tender. Add the broccoli for the last 2 minutes of cooking. Drain, then slice the potatoes into thick pieces.

2 / Meanwhile, place the mixed beans and green beans in a separate pan, cover with water and bring to the boil. Reduce the heat and simmer for 3 minutes or until the green beans are tender. Drain and set aside in the pan.

3 / Preheat the grill (broiler) to medium-high.

4 / Gently heat 1 tablespoon of the oil in an ovenproof frying pan (skillet) over a low heat. Add the garlic and cook for 1 minute, then add the potatoes and broccoli and stir to coat in the oil.

5 / Lightly beat the eggs in a bowl and pour over the potato and broccoli mixture. Cook for 3–5 minutes until the bottom of the frittata is almost set. Scatter the ricotta over the frittata, then pop the pan under the grill for 8–10 minutes or until the frittata is cooked in the middle.

6 / Meanwhile, mix the remaining olive oil with the cider vinegar in a small bowl and pour over the beans. Stir in the chopped basil and season to taste with freshly ground black pepper.

7 / Slice the frittata into 4 equal slices and serve with the bean salad.

options
For a dairy-free version, omit the ricotta and sprinkle with nutritional yeast flakes once the frittata is cooked.

In place of ricotta, use feta or goat's cheese. Cow's dairy can be inflammatory for some people, so using anti-inflammatory goat or sheep dairy (e.g. in feta) can be helpful.

avocado and black bean eggs

Black beans are a staple food in Central and South America. Like many other beans, they are a great source of protein, fibre and folate. Avocados are also an excellent source of fibre, as well as being rich in antioxidants and healthy monounsaturated fat.

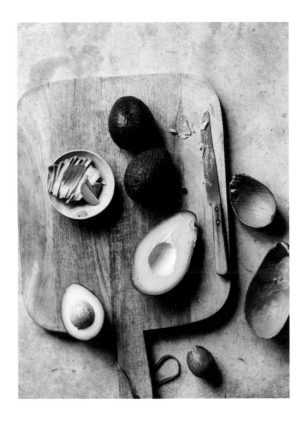

Serves 4

1 Tbsp olive oil

2 garlic cloves, finely sliced

4 medium or large eggs

2 x 400g (14oz) cans black beans, drained

400g (14oz) cherry tomatoes

2 tsp paprika

2 avocados, preferably Hass, flesh removed and sliced

1 lime, quartered

freshly ground black pepper

df gf

options
For a vegan option, omit the eggs and replace with pinto beans.

tips
Try spicing it up by adding finely sliced red chilli – it gives a delicious kick.

1 / Gently heat the olive oil in a large frying pan (skillet) over a low heat. Add the garlic and cook until softened, then crack in the eggs on different sides of the pan. Cook until almost set, then add the beans and tomatoes, sprinkle with the paprika and gently heat through.

2 / Remove from the heat and place the sliced avocado on top of the beans and tomatoes. Squeeze the juice of 1 lime wedge onto each egg and season to taste with freshly ground pepper.

3 / Serve from the pan at the table.

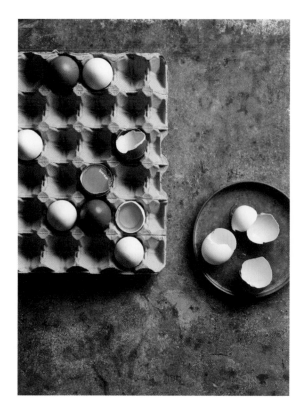

grain-free spinach and parmesan quiche

This flour-free quiche is completely gluten-free, and is incredibly quick and easy to make – literally whisk all the ingredients together and pop in the oven!

Serves 4

2 tsp olive oil

4 medium or large eggs

125ml (4fl oz/½ cup) crème fraîche

100g (3½oz/1½ cups) finely grated Parmesan

large handful of spinach, roughly chopped

2 garlic cloves, crushed

freshly ground black pepper

To serve:
green salad

Homemade Vinaigrette (see page 198)

gf

tips
This is also delicious served with Crunchy Coleslaw (see page 193).

1 / Preheat the oven to 180°C (350°F/gas 4) and grease an ovenproof dish with the olive oil.

2 / In a large bowl, whisk the eggs and crème fraîche together, then stir in the Parmesan, spinach and garlic. Pour the egg mixture into the prepared dish and bake in the oven for 20–25 minutes until cooked through.

3 / Season to taste with freshly ground black pepper.

4 / Serve with a green salad dressed with vinaigrette.

broccoli and turmeric hash

This is a wonderful anti-inflammatory recipe that your gut will absolutely love. Broccoli is a rich source of fibre, as well as of multiple vitamins and minerals, including vitamin C, which helps to support healthy immune response. Broccoli also provides powerful antioxidants that may aid in supporting cells and tissues throughout your body. In addition, turmeric – and particularly its most active compound, curcumin – has many evidence-based health benefits – it is a potent antioxidant and anti-inflammatory.

Serves 4

2 tsp olive oil

1 red onion, chopped

1 small head of broccoli, chopped into small pieces

1 tsp ground turmeric

4 large eggs

2 avocados, preferably Hass, flesh removed and chopped

freshly ground black pepper

df gf

1 / Gently heat the oil in a frying pan (skillet) over a low heat. Add the red onion and broccoli and sauté for about 5 minutes. Add the turmeric, crack in the eggs, and combine with the onion and broccoli. Cook until the egg is firm, then add the avocado and stir through, breaking the mixture up a little.

2 / Serve, seasoned to taste with freshly ground black pepper.

options
For a vegan option, replace the eggs with 100g (3½oz) silken tofu.

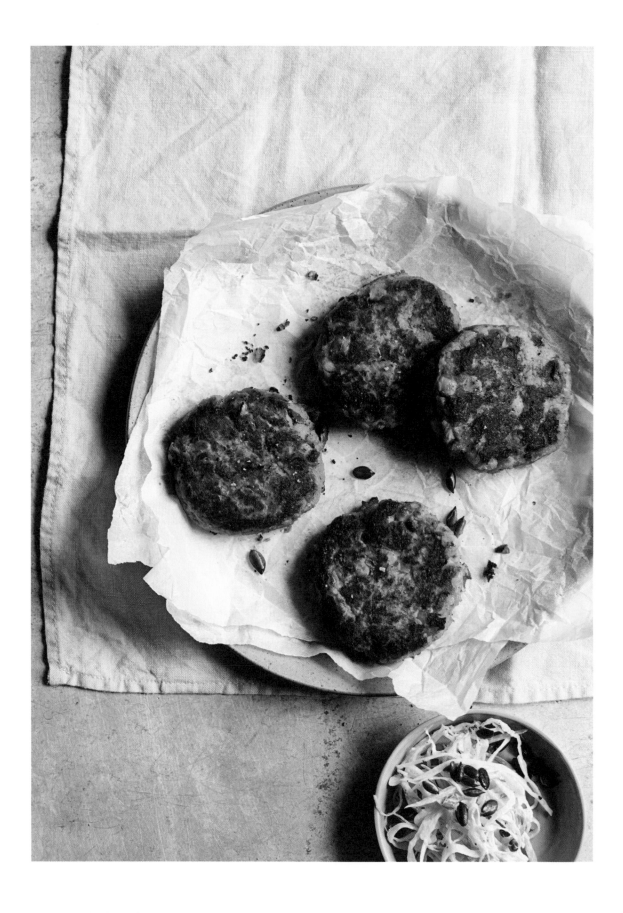

chickpea and cumin burgers

Chickpeas, also known as garbanzo beans, are a great source of fibre and protein. Also, many scientific studies have shown that beans and legumes can help reduce weight, risk factors for heart disease and potentially even the risk of cancer, especially when they replace red meat in the diet.

Serves 4

2 Tbsp olive oil

1 white onion, chopped

1 carrot, grated

1 tsp ground cumin

1 tsp curry powder

1 tsp ground turmeric

1 x 400g (14oz) can chickpeas (garbanzo beans), drained

1 egg, whisked

zest and juice of 1 lemon

freshly ground black pepper

1 / Heat 1 tablespoon of the olive oil in a frying pan (skillet) over a medium heat. Add the onion and grated carrot and cook for 5 minutes. Add the spices, stir well, and cook for 3 minutes, then transfer the mixture to a mixing bowl and let cool.

2 / Add the chickpeas and the egg to the mixing bowl and use a hand-held blender to thoroughly combine the mixture. Add the lemon zest and juice, mix well, then season with freshly ground black pepper. Shape the mixture into 4 patties and place in the fridge for 30 minutes to firm up.

3 / When ready to cook, heat the remaining tablespoon of olive oil in a frying pan over a medium heat. Add the burgers and cook for 6 minutes on each side, turning once during cooking.

options
For a vegan option, replace the egg with 1 Tbsp flax seeds (linseeds) or chia seeds, or 1 Tbsp coconut yoghurt.

tips
Serve these burgers with Crunchy Coleslaw (see page 193).

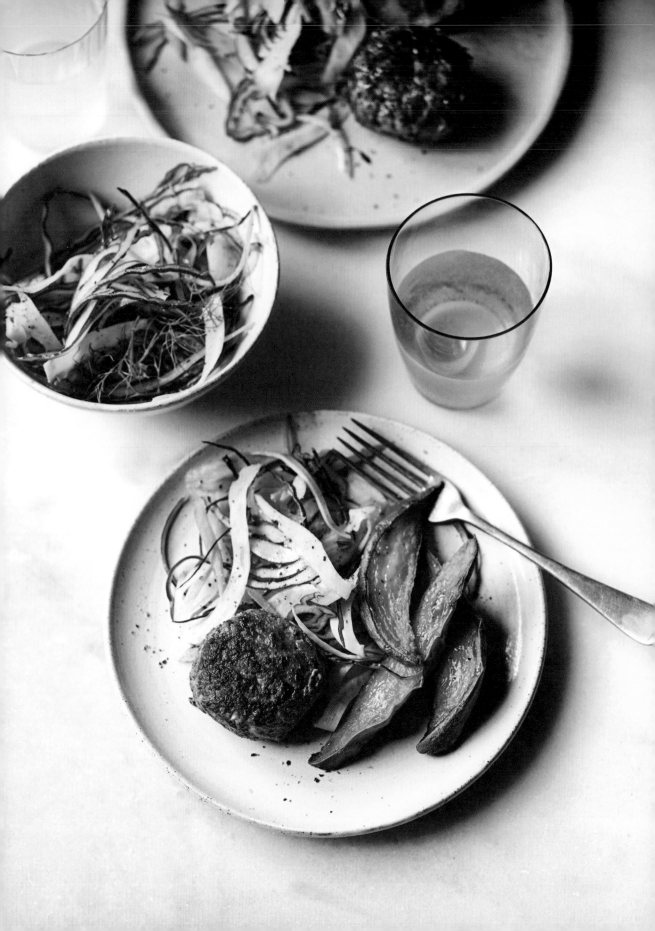

turkey burgers

Turkey is rich in protein and an excellent source of numerous vitamins and minerals, including B vitamins and selenium, zinc and phosphorus, which are essential to health.

Serves 4

1 white onion, chopped

2 garlic cloves, crushed

2 tsp dried mixed herbs

large handful of fresh coriander (cilantro)

zest of 1 lime

½ tsp sea salt (kosher salt)

freshly ground black pepper

4 Tbsp olive oil

400g (14oz) minced (ground) turkey

To serve:
Crunchy Coleslaw (see page 193)

Sweet Potato Wedges (see page 192)

df gf

1 / Place the onion, garlic, mixed herbs, coriander, lime zest, salt, some pepper and 1 tablespoon of the oil into a blender or food processor and blitz to combine.

2 / Transfer the mixture to a mixing bowl, add the turkey and mix well (you may find this easier using your hands). Shape the mixture into 6–8 patties and place in the fridge for 25 minutes to firm up.

3 / Heat the remaining 3 tablespoons of oil in a large frying pan (skillet) over a medium heat. Add the burgers and cook for 6–8 minutes on each side, turning once, until they are browned and cooked through in the middle.

4 / Serve with coleslaw and sweet potato wedges.

satay tofu skewers

Tofu is a good source of protein and contains all nine essential amino acids. It is also a valuable plant source of iron and calcium and the minerals manganese and phosphorous. Tofu also contains magnesium, copper, zinc and vitamin B1.

Serves 4

6 Tbsp peanut butter

2 tsp soy sauce

2 limes: 1 juiced; 1 cut into wedges

400g (14oz) firm tofu, cut into chunks

2 Tbsp peanuts, roasted

You will need 8 skewers

df vg

1 / In a small bowl, combine the peanut butter, soy sauce and lime juice with 75ml (2½fl oz/⅓ cup) water.

2 / Pour half of the satay sauce mixture into a roasting tin (pan), add the tofu and coat well. Leave to marinate for at least 30 minutes, if possible (don't worry if you don't have time – it's not essential).

3 / Meanwhile, preheat the grill (broiler) to high.

4 / Thread the chunks of marinated tofu onto skewers and place on a baking sheet. Place under the grill and cook the skewers for 4–5 minutes, turning until browned on all sides.

5 / Remove from the heat and drizzle the remaining satay sauce over the tofu. Sprinkle over the peanuts and serve with the lime wedges.

options
For a gluten-free option, use tamari in place of the soy sauce.

tips
I have used almond butter when I didn't have any peanut butter and it worked a treat – so, do experiment with different nut butters.

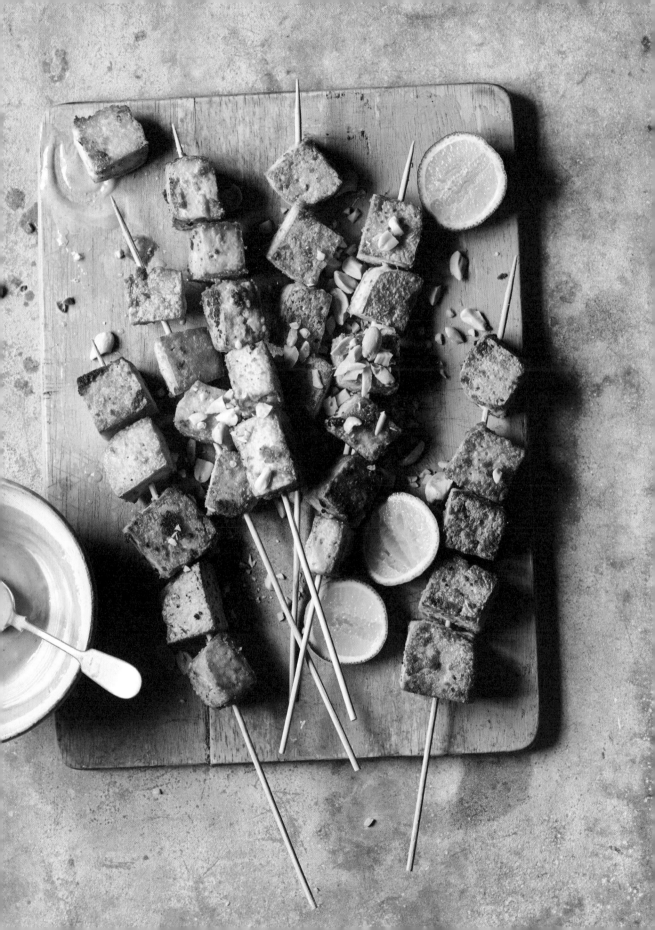

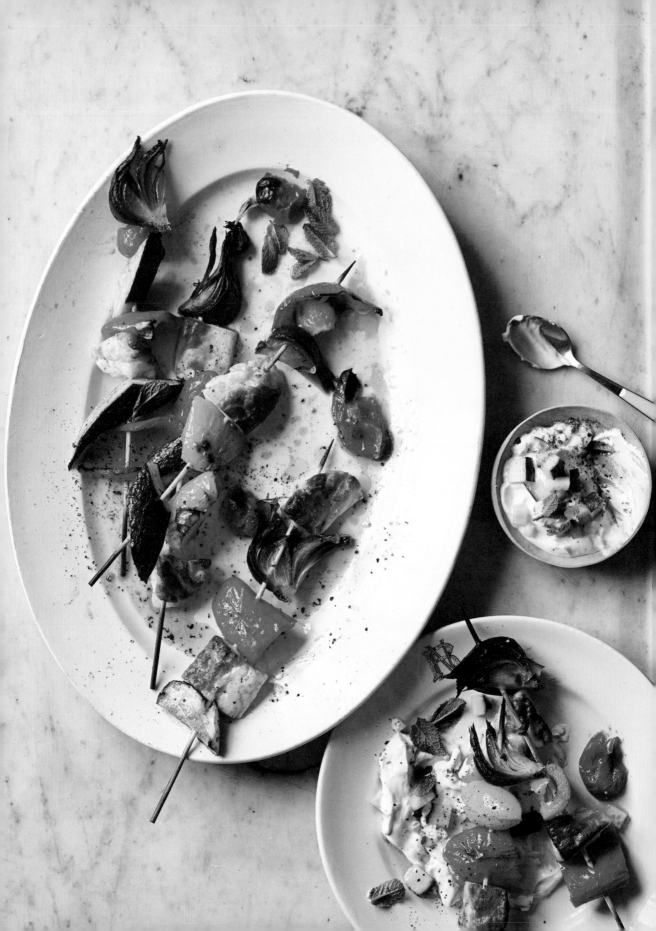

halloumi kebabs with raita

Halloumi is high in protein, making it a good vegetarian option. It is an excellent source of calcium, providing 70 per cent of the adult recommended daily allowance in one portion. It also contains zinc, selenium, magnesium, vitamin A and many of the B vitamins. However, it is high in salt and saturated fat, so enjoy it in moderation.

Serves 4

250g (9oz) halloumi, cut into 16 cubes

1 large red onion, cut into bite-size pieces

1 yellow (bell) pepper, cut into bite-size pieces

1 red (bell) pepper, deseeded and cut into bite-size pieces

2 courgettes (zucchini), halved and cut into bite-size wedges

16 cherry tomatoes

4 Tbsp olive oil

2 tsp paprika

For the raita:
250ml (8fl oz/generous 1 cup) organic Greek yoghurt

½ cucumber, grated or diced

1 garlic clove, crushed

3cm (1in) piece of fresh root ginger, grated

3–4 mint leaves, chopped

juice of ½ lime

½ tsp garam masala

pinch of sea salt (kosher salt)

freshly ground black pepper

You will need 8 skewers

1 / Preheat the grill (broiler) to high.

2 / Place the halloumi, onion, peppers, courgettes and tomatoes in a large mixing bowl. Add the olive oil and make sure everything is well coated with the oil. Alternately thread the halloumi and vegetables onto the skewers and sprinkle with the paprika.

3 / Grill (broil) for about 5 minutes, turning frequently until coloured on all sides.

4 / Meanwhile, add all the ingredients for the raita to a mixing bowl. Mix well and adjust the seasoning to taste.

5 / Serve immediately.

tips
If you don't have time to make the raita, you can just use Greek yoghurt or thick live natural (plain) yoghurt as a dipping sauce. As well as a great dressing for these kebabs, raita is a perfect accompaniment to a curry.

beetroot, spinach and goat's cheese couscous

Once considered a North African delicacy, couscous is now eaten all over the world. One of the most important nutrients in couscous is selenium, which is an essential mineral with many health benefits. It's a powerful antioxidant that helps your body repair damaged cells and reduces inflammation, thus decreasing oxidative stress, which in turn promotes immunity. About 150g (5½oz/scant 1 cup) of couscous contains more than 60 per cent of the recommended daily intake of selenium. Combined with beetroot (beets) and goat's cheese, this dish packs a nutritional punch.

Serves 4

zest and juice of 1 lemon

zest and juice of 2 oranges

280g (10oz/1¾ cups) couscous

150g (5½oz) goat's cheese, crumbled

80g (3oz/⅔ cup) walnuts, chopped

4 small beetroot (beets), cooked and cut into small chunks

freshly ground black pepper

To serve:
4 handfuls of baby spinach

Homemade Vinaigrette
(see page 198)

1 / Bring 200ml (7fl oz/scant 1 cup) water to the boil in a saucepan. Reduce the heat to medium, add the lemon and orange zests and juices and simmer for 2 minutes.

2 / Put the couscous into a large bowl and pour over the hot infused water. Mix well, cover the bowl with a plate, and let rest for 5–6 minutes until the liquid is absorbed.

3 / Fluff up the couscous with a fork, then add the goat's cheese, walnuts and beetroot. Season with freshly ground black pepper.

4 / When you are ready to eat, toss the baby spinach leaves through and serve with vinaigrette.

options
For a gluten-free option, replace the couscous with quinoa, which is a great plant-based protein source.

For a vegan or dairy-free option, replace the goat's cheese with chia seeds and sprinkle with nutritional yeast.

tips
This is a great recipe to double up, as you can then enjoy it the next day as a lunchbox lunch. If you leave tossing the baby spinach through to the last minute (keep it on top of the couscous), this will make sure it doesn't go soggy if you are transporting it to work with you.

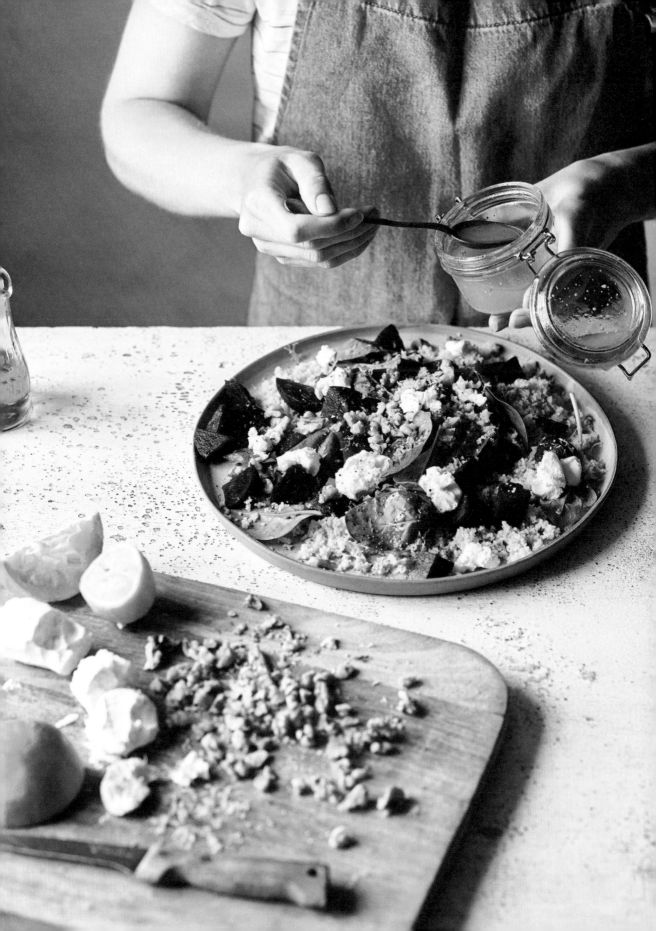

wild salmon veggie bowl

This makes a quick, delicious, protein-packed lunch that is low-calorie, rich in beneficial omega-3 fats and is dairy- and gluten-free, too. I always try to use wild salmon rather than farmed salmon as it is higher in minerals, such as iron, zinc and potassium. Also, farmed salmon contains up to three times more saturated fat than wild salmon.

Serves 4

2 small courgettes (zucchini)

4 carrots

3 beetroot (beets), cooked and diced

2 red onions, finely chopped

4 Tbsp balsamic vinegar

small bunch of fresh dill, chopped

500g (1lb 2oz) poached salmon or canned wild salmon

4 Tbsp capers, rinsed

freshly ground black pepper

df gf

1 / Use a spiralizer or julienne peeler to shred the courgettes and carrots into long strips, and divide among 4 plates or shallow bowls.

2 / In a bowl, combine the cooked beetroot, red onions, balsamic vinegar and dill. Divide the mixture among the plates, placing it on top of the courgettes and carrots.

3 / Flake the salmon with a fork, then scatter it over the vegetables. Sprinkle with the capers and season to taste with freshly ground black pepper.

options
For a vegan option, replace the salmon with smoked tofu.

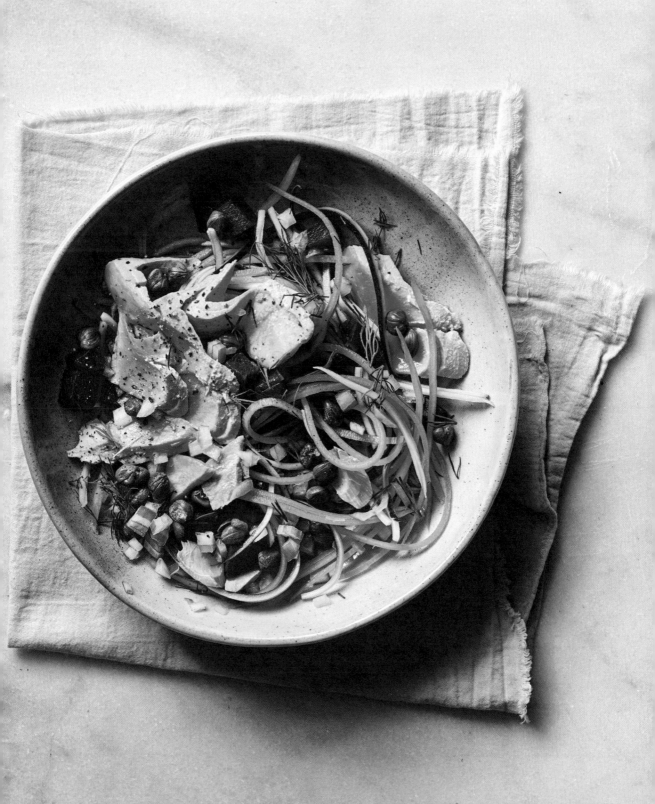

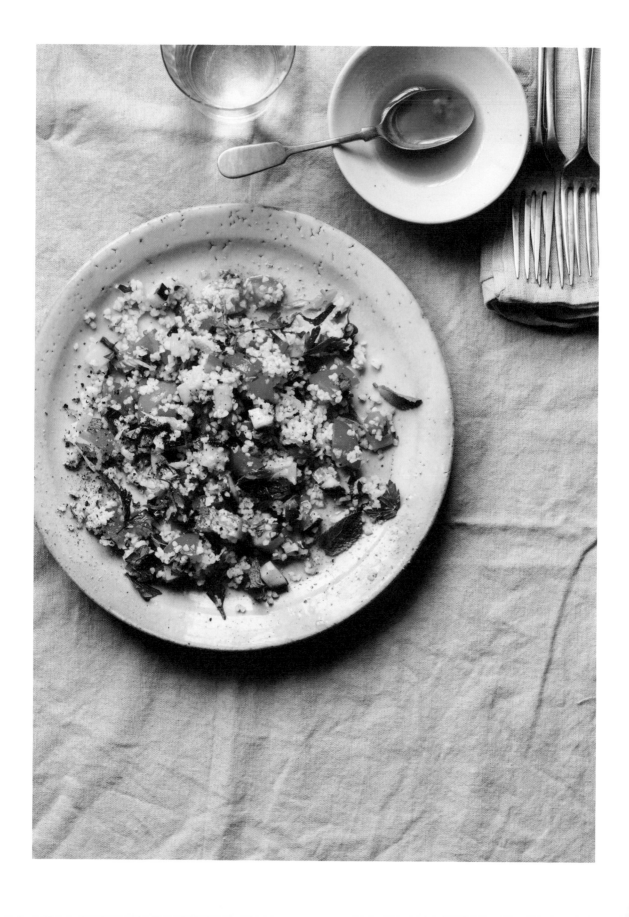

minty bulgur tabbouleh

Bulgur is a whole grain made from cracked wheat. It's packed with vitamins, minerals and fibre. Fibre is incredibly important for our health as it has been shown to improve digestion and gut health, as well as reducing chronic disease risk and promoting weight loss.

Serves 4

180g (1⅓oz/1½ cups) bulgur wheat

250g (9oz) ripe tomatoes, finely chopped

1 small cucumber, finely diced

4 spring onions (scallions), finely sliced

juice of 2 lemons

½ tsp freshly ground black pepper

½ tsp ground nutmeg

½ tsp ground ginger

large handful of parsley, stalks removed, finely chopped

small handful of mint leaves, finely chopped

75ml (2½fl oz/⅓ cup) olive oil

pinch of sea salt (kosher salt)

For the dressing:
4 Tbsp olive oil

2 Tbsp lemon juice

1 garlic clove, crushed

½ tsp cayenne pepper

sea salt (kosher salt) and freshly ground black pepper

1 / Place the bulgur wheat in a large saucepan and cover with water or stock, according to the instructions on the packet. Bring to the boil, then reduce the heat and gently simmer for 10 minutes, adding more water if required. Remove from the heat, cover and set aside for 12–15 minutes.

2 / Add the tomatoes, cucumber and spring onions to the bulgur wheat, along with three-quarters of the lemon juice. Combine the black pepper, nutmeg and ginger together, then add 1 teaspoon of the mixed spices to the bulgur wheat. Add the parsley, mint, olive oil and the remaining lemon juice, then season with sea salt and toss thoroughly.

3 / Meanwhile, whisk all the dressing ingredients together in a bowl, seasoning with salt and black pepper to taste.

4 / Stir the dressing through the salad just before serving.

options
For a gluten-free option, replace the bulgur wheat with quinoa.

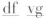

homemade hummus with spicy flax seed crackers

These crackers are nutrient dense and ultra-versatile. They can be enjoyed not only with hummus, they also work really well with goat's cheese, feta, Manchego or even spread with a nut butter (see page 199). A silicone baking sheet or tray is required for this recipe.

Serves 4

For the crackers:
1 tsp olive oil

½ yellow, orange or red (bell) pepper

100g (3½oz/¾cup) flax seeds (linseeds)

30g (1oz/⅓ cup) ground almonds

30g (1oz/2 Tbsp) chia seeds

¼ tsp chilli powder

2 tsp tomato purée (paste) or passata

For the hummus:
1 x 400g (14oz) can chickpeas (garbanzo beans), drained and rinsed

1 garlic clove, crushed

1 Tbsp tahini

60ml (2¼fl oz/¼ cup) extra-virgin olive oil

½ tsp ground cumin

juice of 1 lemon

pinch of sea salt (kosher salt)

freshly ground black pepper

df gf vg

1 / First, make the crackers. Preheat the oven to 140°C (275°F/gas 1).

2 / Brush the pepper with the olive oil, place on a baking sheet and pop in the oven for 15–20 minutes, or until softened. Remove from the oven and set aside to cool.

3 / Meanwhile, combine the flax seeds, ground almonds, chia seeds, chilli powder and tomato purée or passata in a food processor or blender along with 25ml (1fl oz/2 Tbsp) water and blitz.

4 / Remove the seeds from the cooled red pepper and roughly chop. Add the pepper to the mixture in the food processor and blitz for 30 seconds. If the mixture crumbles or looks a little dry, then add 1 teaspoon of water.

5 / Turn the mixture out onto the work surface and use a rolling pin to roll it as thin as possible, about 5mm (¼in), then transfer to a silicone baking sheet or tray. Score into squares and bake for about 40 minutes, swivelling the baking sheet a couple of times during baking in case your oven has any hotspots.

6 / Remove the crackers from the oven once golden and crisp, and split into squares.

7 / Meanwhile, make the hummus. Combine the chickpeas, garlic, tahini, oil, cumin and lemon juice in a food processor or blender along with 50ml (2fl oz/scant ¼ cup) water. Blitz for 2–3 minutes, or until smooth. Add the salt and blitz for a further 30 seconds, then season to taste with freshly ground black pepper.

8 / Serve the hummus with the crackers.

option
Tahini is crushed sesame seeds. I have made the hummus before with unsalted almond butter when I didn't have any tahini and it worked really well!

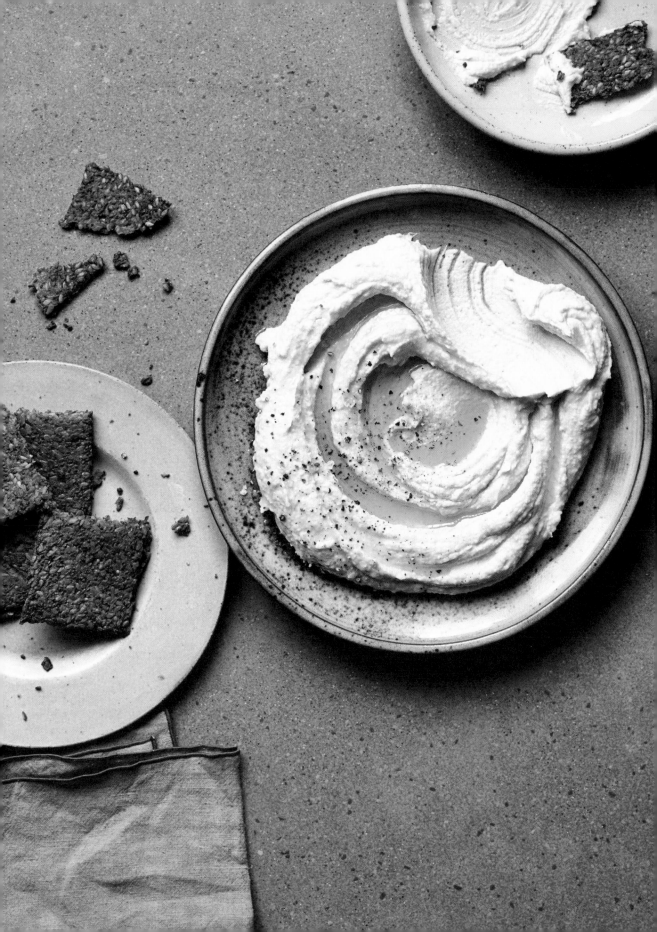

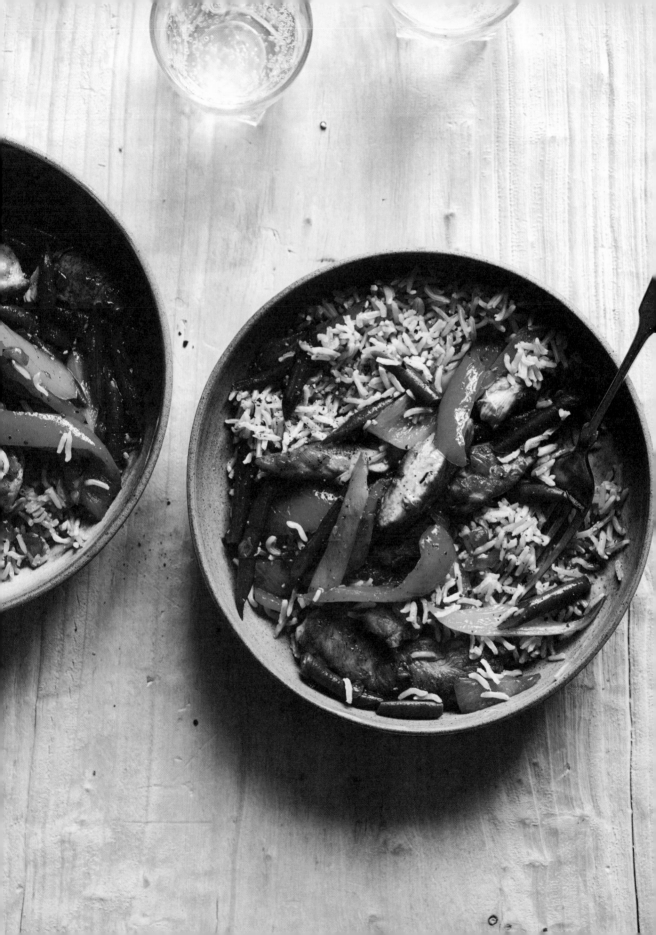

coconut chicken and green bean stir-fry

Chicken is high in protein and lower in fat than other animal sources, such as beef, particularly the breast meat. In addition, chicken is a great source of iron, zinc, selenium and B vitamins.

Serves 4

4 chicken breasts, thinly sliced

4 tsp paprika

2 Tbsp coconut oil (see Tip)

400g (14oz) mixed (bell) peppers, deseeded and chopped

1 white onion, chopped

2 garlic cloves, chopped

150g (5½oz) green beans, thinly sliced

1–2 Tbsp soy sauce

freshly ground black pepper

To serve:
200g (7oz/1 cup) brown rice or
1 x recipe quantity Cauliflower Rice
(see page 192)

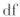

1 / Season the chicken with the paprika and set aside.

2 / Heat the coconut oil in a sauté pan over a medium heat, then add the mixed peppers, onion and garlic and cook for 5 minutes. Increase the heat, add the seasoned chicken and green beans and cook for 8–10 minutes, or until the chicken is cooked through. Add the soy sauce 2 minutes before the end of cooking.

3 / Meanwhile, if serving with brown rice, bring a pan of water to the boil and cook the rice according to the packet instructions. If serving with cauliflower rice, follow the instructions on page 192.

4 / Season the stir-fry with freshly ground black pepper and serve with brown rice or cauliflower rice.

options

For a vegan option, replace the chicken with 250g (9oz) silken tofu.

For a gluten-free option, use tamari in place of the soy sauce.

tips

Make your own Coconut Oil to use in this recipe (see page 200).

aubergine and tomato hake

Aubergine, also known as eggplant, is my favourite vegetable and it works really well in this dish with hake. This is really straightforward and quick to bring together, making it an ideal supper when you are short on time.

Serves 4

1 Tbsp olive oil

1 onion, finely chopped

250g (9oz) aubergine (eggplant), chopped

200g (7oz/generous 1 cup) chopped tomatoes

1 garlic clove, crushed

½ tsp paprika

4 large basil leaves, plus a few extra for sprinkling

600g (1lb 5oz) hake fillets

pinch of sea salt (kosher salt)

freshly ground black pepper

df gf

1 / Heat the olive oil in a large frying pan (skillet) over a low–medium heat. Add the onion and aubergine and cook for 4 minutes, then cover with a lid and let the vegetables steam-fry in their own juices for 5–6 minutes. Stir in the tomatoes, garlic and paprika and cook for 8 minutes, stirring, until the aubergine is soft. Add the basil leaves, then nestle the fish in the sauce, cover the pan and cook for 8–10 minutes, or until the fish is cooked through.

2 / Serve, seasoned with a pinch of sea salt and freshly ground black pepper to taste.

tips
If you don't have fresh tomatoes, use canned chopped tomatoes.

You can use any white fish in this recipe in place of hake.

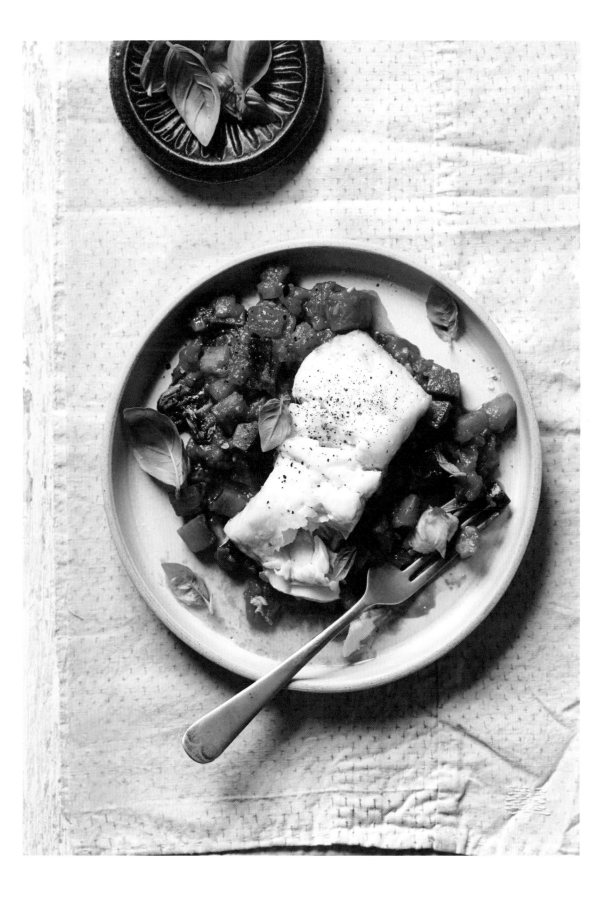

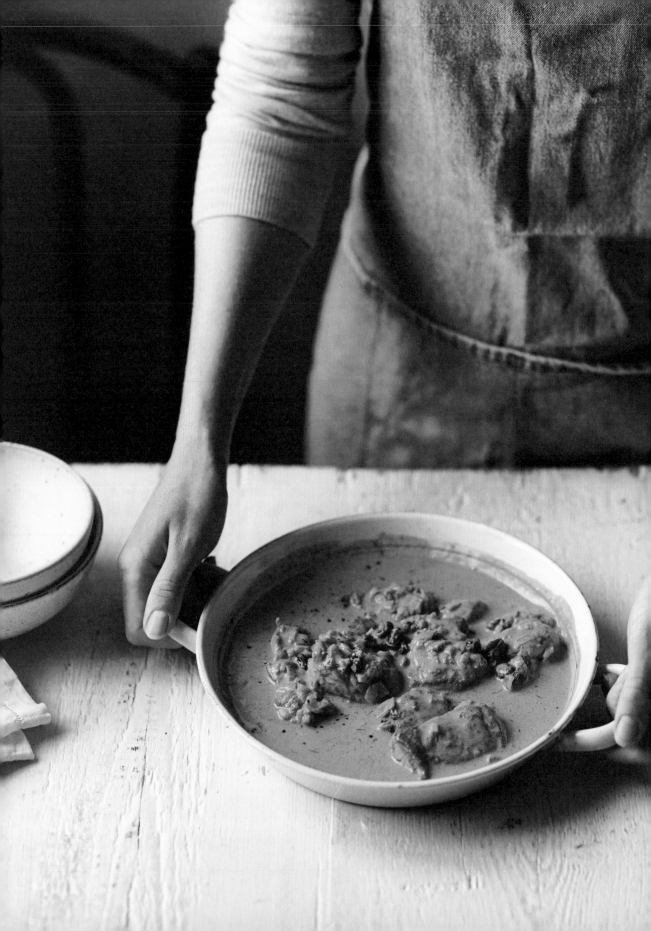

chicken curry

Dark chicken meat is higher in vitamins A and D than the white meat. These vitamins play an important role in supporting gut health and immune function, which is why I tend to make this recipe with chicken thighs.

Serves 4

2 Tbsp olive oil

500g (1lb 2 oz) skinless and boneless chicken thighs, chopped into large chunks

1 white onion, chopped

2 garlic cloves, crushed

1 Tbsp medium curry powder

1 tsp ground turmeric

1 tsp ground cardamom

1 Tbsp tomato purée (paste)

200ml (7fl oz/scant 1 cup) coconut yoghurt or organic Greek yoghurt

200ml (7fl oz/scant 1 cup) chicken stock (bouillon)

handful of raisins

freshly ground black pepper

To serve:
Cauliflower Rice (see page 192)

1 / Heat the oil in a saucepan over a medium heat. Add the chicken thighs and cook until lightly browned all over, then remove to a plate and set aside.

2 / Add the onion, garlic and curry powder to the same pan and sweat for 5 minutes until the onion starts to soften. Stir in the turmeric and cardamom and cook for a further 4–5 minutes, then add the chicken back to the pan along with the tomato purée. Add the yoghurt and stock gradually, stirring well to incorporate, then reduce the heat and simmer for 30 minutes, stirring occasionally and adding more water if it starts to look dry. Add the raisins and continue to simmer for a further 15 minutes.

3 / Meanwhile, prepare the cauliflower rice according to the instructions on page 192.

4 / Season the curry to taste with freshly ground black pepper and serve with the cauliflower rice.

options
For a dairy-free option, use coconut yoghurt instead of Greek yoghurt.

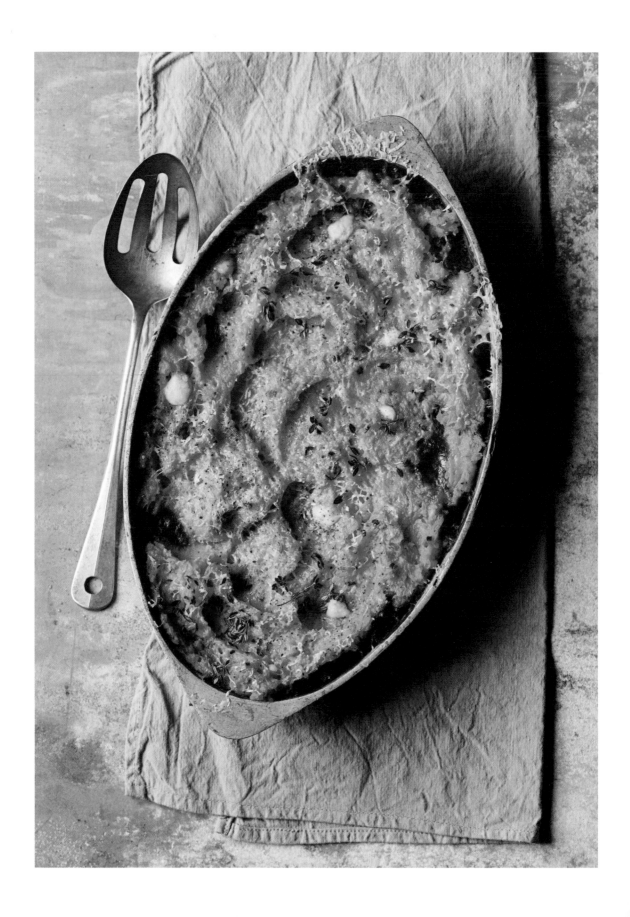

veggie cottage pie with sweet potato mash

I love this plant-based cottage pie as it is packed with nutrients. I always make it with lentils, which are made up of over 25 per cent of protein and are thus a brilliant plant-based alternative to meat. Lentils also contain lots of other important nutrients that support our health, including magnesium, zinc, potassium, iron and B vitamins. I use sweet potatoes over white potatoes in this dish, as they are rich in fibre, vitamins and minerals, and are high in antioxidants that help protect our bodies from free radical damage and chronic disease. Also, the fibre and antioxidants in sweet potatoes promote the growth of beneficial gut bacteria and promote a healthy gut.

Serves 4

2 Tbsp olive oil

1 large onion, sliced

2 large carrots, diced

small bunch of fresh thyme, chopped

150ml (5fl oz/⅔ cup) red wine, vegan if necessary

1 x 400g (14oz) can chopped tomatoes

2 low-salt vegetable stock (bouillon) cubes

1 x 400g (14oz) can black Beluga lentils

1kg (2lb 3oz) sweet potatoes, peeled and cut into chunks

1 tsp ground nutmeg

100g (3½oz/generous 1 cup) grated vegan cheddar

freshly ground black pepper

df gf vg

1 / Gently heat the olive oil in a saucepan over a low heat. Add the onion and sweat for 5 minutes until softened, then add the carrots and most of the chopped thyme, reserving a little for sprinkling over later. Add the wine, 50ml (2fl oz/scant ¼ cup) water and the tomatoes, and crumble in the stock cubes. Simmer for 10–12 minutes. Add the lentils and their canning liquid, cover and simmer for a further 12 minutes until the lentils are pulpy.

2 / Meanwhile, preheat the oven to 180°C (350°F/gas 4).

3 / Bring a large saucepan of water to the boil, add the sweet potatoes and cook for 15 minutes until tender. Drain and mash the potatoes and sprinkle over the nutmeg.

4 / Transfer the cooked lentils to an ovenproof dish, top with the sweet potato mash and scatter over the cheese and the reserved thyme. Pop in the oven and cook for 30 minutes until golden and cooked though. Season to taste with freshly ground black pepper.

options

If you are not vegan or dairy-free, you can use a mature cheddar in place of the vegan cheese.

If you don't drink alcohol, you can omit the wine and replace with vegetable stock (bouillon).

tips

You can use any kind of lentils in this dish – I tend to use black Beluga lentils as they have a full-bodied flavour and work really well in hearty dishes such as this or casseroles.

This is a great dish to cook in batches and pop in the freezer (it will keep for up to a month in the freezer). Alternatively, you can keep it covered in the fridge for 2 days.

spicy bulgur with roasted peppers

This is a very quick dish that you can make as a supper when you are short on time. Bulgur wheat is a whole grain that has been parboiled, which allows it to be cooked more quickly while retaining a fairly high content of fibre. This dish tastes delicious with the spices and the fresh coriander (cilantro) – a wonderful herb that is a great natural detoxifier and is anti-inflammatory.

Serves 4

200g (7oz/scant 1¼ cups) bulgur wheat

250ml (8fl oz/1 cup) vegetable stock (bouillon), or as needed

1 Tbsp olive oil

½ tsp ground cumin

½ tsp ground cinnamon

zest and juice of 1 lemon

1 x 400g (14oz) can chickpeas (garbanzo beans), drained

1 red or white onion, finely diced

small jar (170g/6oz) roasted (bell) peppers, drained and sliced

small bunch of fresh coriander (cilantro), chopped

freshly ground black pepper

df vg

1 / Place the bulgur wheat in a saucepan and cover with the hot stock, according to the packet instructions. Bring to the boil, then reduce the heat and gently simmer for 10 minutes, adding more water or stock if required. Remove from the heat, cover and set aside for 12–15 minutes.

2 / Meanwhile, mix the olive oil, cumin, cinnamon, lemon zest and juice together in a large mixing bowl. Add the chickpeas, onion, peppers, coriander and finally the bulgur wheat. Mix well and season to taste with freshly ground black pepper.

options
For a gluten-free option replace the bulgur wheat with quinoa.

To roast the pepper yourself, preheat the oven to 220°C (425°F/gas 7). Place 1 red (bell) pepper, halved and deseeded, on a baking sheet and brush with olive oil. Roast for 30 minutes, then remove from the oven and leave to cool. Once cool, remove the skin and cut into slices.

tips
This is a great dish to cook more of and enjoy cold as a lunchbox lunch the next day.

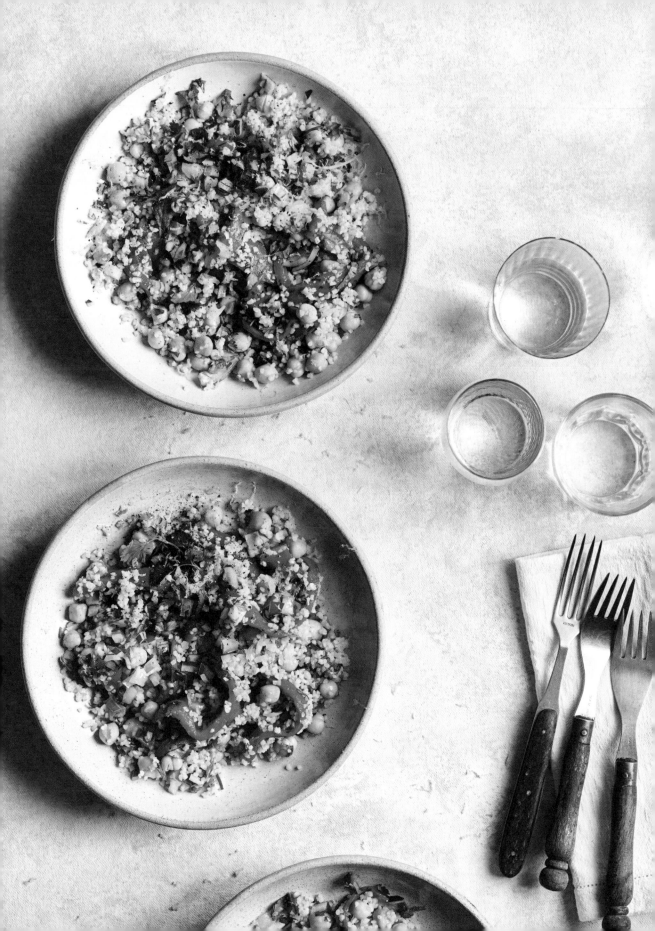

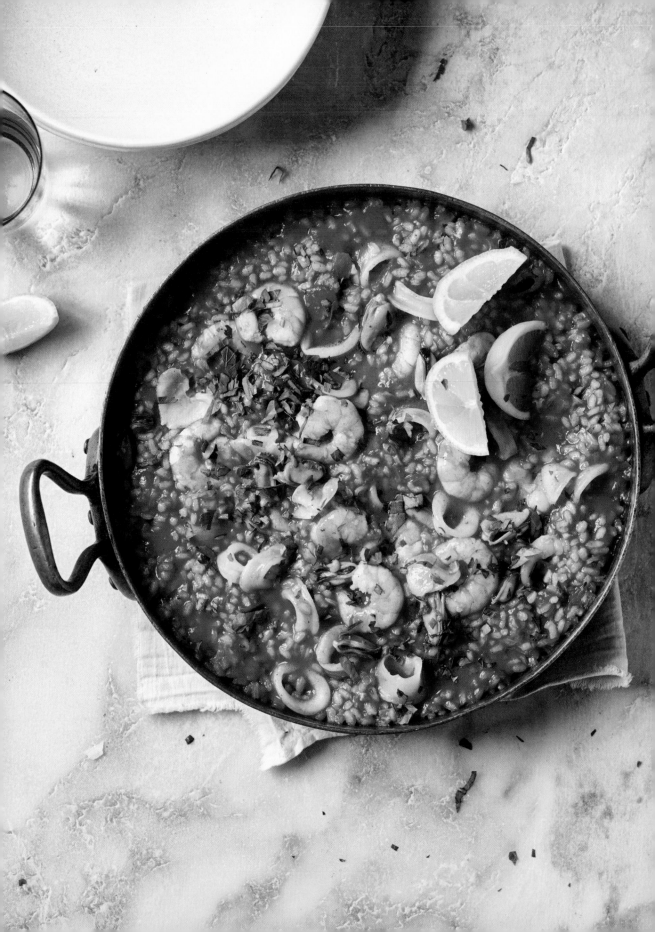

easy peasy paella

Thanks to the addition of the mixed seafood, this paella is packed with zinc, a mineral that's essential for good health. Zinc is required for the functions of over 300 enzymes and is involved in many important processes in your body. It metabolizes nutrients, maintains your immune system and repairs body tissues. As your body doesn't store zinc, you need to eat enough every day to ensure you're meeting your daily requirements, and this paella is a great way to include it in your diet.

Serves 4

1 Tbsp olive oil

1 red onion, chopped

280g (10oz/1½ cups) paella rice

1 tsp chilli powder

1 tsp ground turmeric

1 x 400g (14oz) can chopped tomatoes

2 garlic cloves, crushed

1 litre (34fl oz/4 cups) fish or chicken stock (bouillon)

1 x 450g (1lb) bag frozen seafood mix

juice of 1 lemon

small handful of flat-leaf parsley, chopped

sea salt (kosher salt) and freshly ground black pepper

lemon wedges, to serve

df gf

1 / Gently heat the olive oil in a wok over a low heat. Add the onion and sweat for 5 minutes until softened, then stir in the rice, chilli powder and turmeric and cook for 1 minute. Add the chopped tomatoes, garlic and stock and cook for about 15 minutes, stirring occasionally, until the rice is almost tender. Stir in the seafood mix, cover and simmer for 8 minutes or until the seafood is cooked through and the rice is completely tender.

2 / Remove from the heat, squeeze over the lemon juice and sprinkle with the parsley, then season with salt and pepper and serve with the lemon wedges.

options
For a vegan option, replace the chicken stock with vegetable stock and the seafood mix with black-eyed beans and kidney beans. Also, add extra veggies, such as peas and red, yellow and orange (bell) peppers.

tips
You can substitute with risotto rice if you don't have paella rice, and experiment by using whatever veggies you have to hand.

As a way to get my children to eat more vegetables, I often add in 150g (5½oz/generous 1 cup) frozen peas along with the seafood.

caribbean butternut squash curry

Butternut squash is an excellent source of many vitamins and minerals, including magnesium, potassium and manganese. It is also an abundant source of potent antioxidants, including vitamins C, E and beta-carotene. Antioxidants are vital to our health, as they help to reduce inflammation, which may decrease your risk of several chronic diseases.

Serves 4

3 Tbsp coconut oil (see Tip)

1 white onion, chopped

2 garlic cloves, crushed

3cm (1in) piece of fresh root ginger, peeled and finely grated

1 red chilli, deseeded and finely chopped

1 tsp ground turmeric

1 tsp ground cumin

1 small butternut squash (about 600g/ 1lb 5oz peeled weight), peeled and cut into 3cm (1in) chunks

300ml (10fl oz/1¼ cups) hot vegetable stock (bouillon), or more as needed

200ml (7fl oz/scant 1 cup) organic Greek yoghurt

juice of 1 lime

freshly ground black pepper

To serve:
Cauliflower Rice (see page 192)

lime wedges

gf

1 / Heat the coconut oil in a saucepan over a medium heat. Add the onion, garlic, ginger and chilli and sweat for 5 minutes until they start to soften. Stir in the turmeric and cumin and cook for a further 2 minutes. Add the butternut squash, then pour in the hot stock followed by the yoghurt. Stir to combine, then reduce the heat to low, cover and simmer for 25 minutes or until the squash is just tender, adding more water or stock if required.

2 / Meanwhile, prepare the cauliflower rice according to the instructions on page 192.

3 / Squeeze the lime juice into the curry, season to taste with freshly ground black pepper, and serve with the cauliflower rice and extra lime wedges.

options
For a vegan or dairy-free option, replace the Greek yoghurt with 150ml (5fl oz/⅔ cup) coconut yoghurt.

tips
Make your own Coconut Oil to use in this recipe (see page 200).

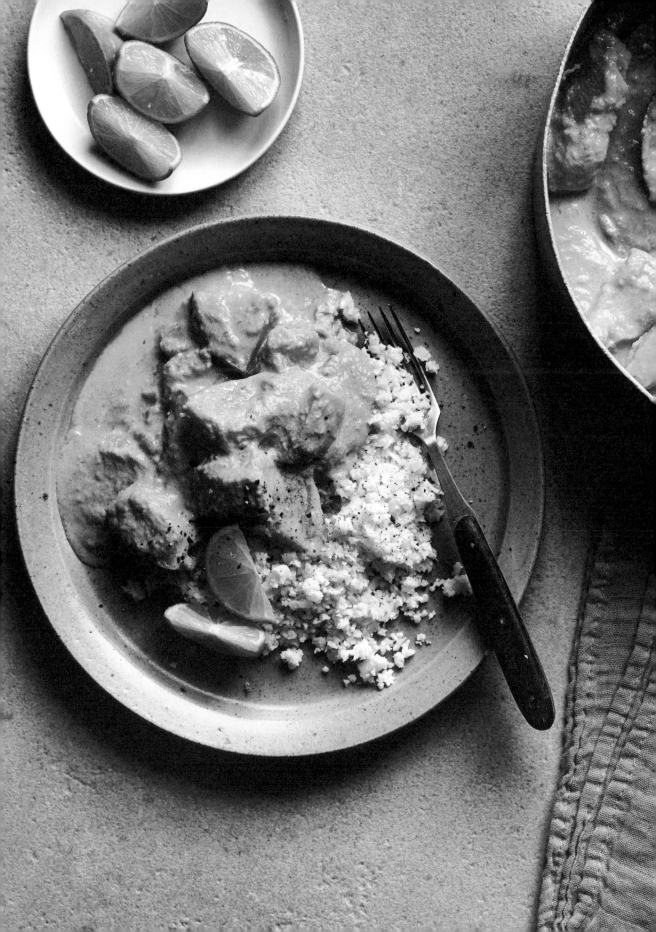

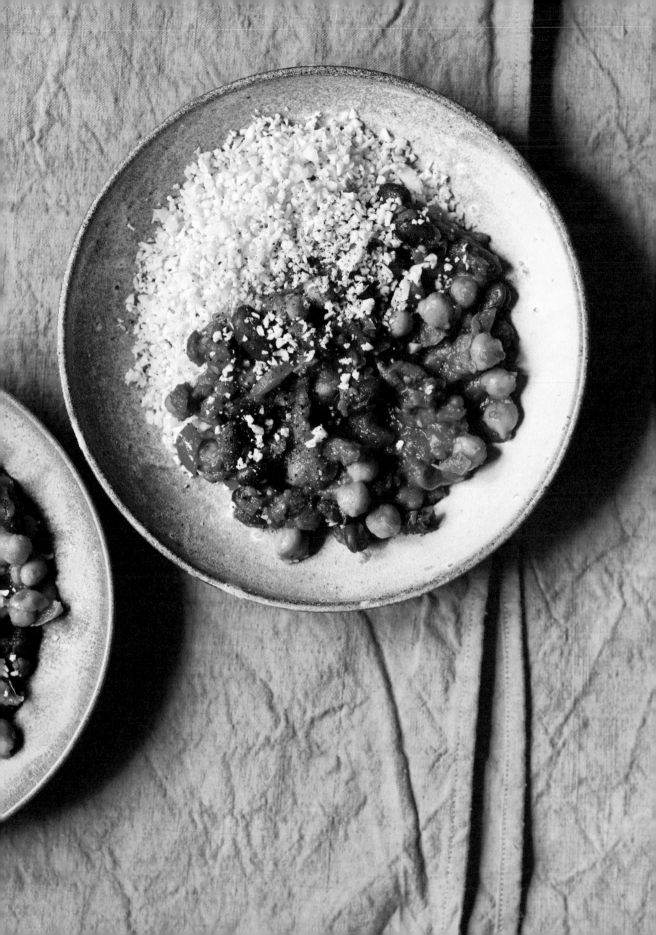

chickpea and bean chilli

Pulses are high in protein, low in fat and low in calories, and they are also a super source of folate and fibre. Chickpeas (garbanzo beans) have also been shown to help reduce blood sugar and cholesterol, and improve gut health. Furthermore, a number of studies have demonstrated that diets containing chickpeas may also help improve bowel function and reduce the number of bad bacteria in the intestines.

Serves 4

3 Tbsp olive oil

1 large onion

1 tsp ground turmeric

1 tsp ground cardamom

1 tsp ground cumin

1 yellow (bell) pepper, deseeded and diced

1 red (bell) pepper, deseeded and diced

2 celery sticks, chopped

2 garlic cloves, crushed

1 tsp dried chilli (red pepper) flakes

2 x 400g (14oz) cans chickpeas (garbanzo beans)

1 x 400g (14oz) can kidney beans

1 x 400g (14oz) can chopped tomatoes

freshly ground black pepper

To serve:
Cauliflower Rice (see page 192)

df gf vg

1 / Gently heat the olive oil in a saucepan over a low heat. Add the onion and sweat for 5 minutes, or until softened. Stir in the turmeric, cardamom and cumin, then add the peppers and celery, and cook for 8–10 minutes. Stir in the garlic, chilli flakes, chickpeas, kidney beans and tomatoes, and simmer for a further 10 minutes.

2 / Meanwhile, prepare the cauliflower rice according to the instructions on page 192.

3 / Season the chilli with freshly ground black pepper to taste, and serve with the cauliflower rice.

tips
This is a really flexible recipe, so you can use whatever veggies and legumes you have to hand – borlotti (cranberry) beans, kidney beans or butter (lima) beans make great alternatives.

chicken biryani with cauliflower rice

This biryani is made with cauliflower rice rather than regular rice, as it is an easy way to help you meet your five-a-day veggie goals, and it is significantly lower in starchy carbs compared to rice, which helps maintain normal blood sugar. Also, it is a great way to get cauliflower, which is a powerful prebiotic, into your diet.

Serves 4

1 cauliflower, grated

2–3 Tbsp coconut oil (see Tip), melted

2 onions, sliced

2 garlic cloves, finely chopped

3cm (1in) piece of fresh root ginger, grated

1 tsp ground turmeric

1 tsp ground cumin

1 tsp ground cardamom

1 tsp ground coriander

½ tsp ground nutmeg

4 chicken breasts, cut into bite-size pieces

80g (3oz/⅔ cup) sultanas (golden raisins)

100ml (3½fl oz/scant ½ cup) chicken stock (bouillon)

handful of fresh coriander (cilantro), chopped

To serve:
homemade raita (see page 119) or Greek yoghurt or natural (plain) live yoghurt

gf

1 / Preheat the oven to 180°C (350°F/gas 4).

2 / Spread the grated cauliflower over a baking sheet and drizzle with 1–2 tablespoons of the coconut oil. Cook in the oven for 10–12 minutes, shaking the baking sheet from time to time to turn the cauliflower. Remove from the oven and set aside.

3 / Meanwhile, heat the remaining 1 tablespoon of coconut oil in a large saucepan over a low heat. Add the onions, garlic, ginger and spices, and cook, stirring, for 5 minutes, or until the onions are softened and golden. Add the chicken and cook for 10 minutes until the chicken is cooked through. Tip in the cauliflower rice, sultanas and stock, then reduce the heat, cover and simmer for 10 minutes.

4 / Sprinkle with the coriander, and serve with raita, or a dollop of Greek or natural (plain) live yoghurt.

options
For a vegan option, replace the chicken breasts with a 400g (14oz) can of lentils or chickpeas (garbanzo beans), and use vegetable stock in place of the chicken stock. Serve with coconut yoghurt.

tips
Make your own Coconut Oil to use in this recipe (see page 200).

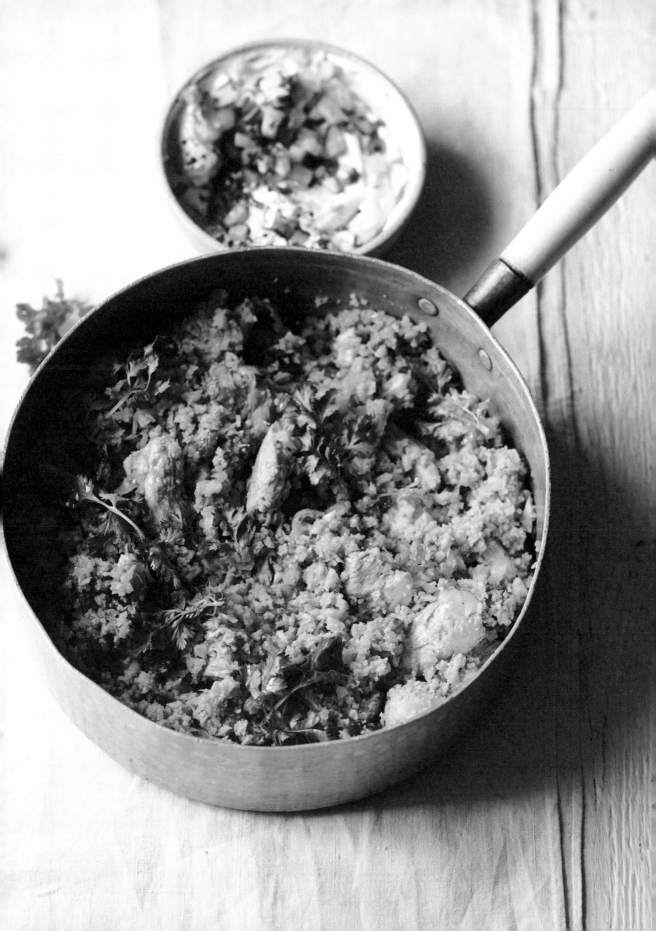

salmon fish cakes with garlic aïoli

Salmon is a fantastic source of several B vitamins, which are required for energy production, promoting optimal heart and brain health, and regulating inflammation. Like other fatty fish, salmon can help to reduce inflammation, which may improve symptoms in individuals with inflammatory conditions, and also decrease the risk of numerous diseases.

Serves 4

4 wild salmon fillets, skinned and cut into chunks

1 Tbsp mayonnaise (see Tip)

2 onions, finely chopped

1 red (bell) pepper, deseeded and finely chopped

1 Tbsp finely chopped dill

2 eggs

4 tsp chia seeds

pinch of sea salt (kosher salt)

1 Tbsp olive oil

For the garlic aïoli:
2 Tbsp avocado oil

½ tsp Dijon mustard

juice of ½ lemon

1 garlic clove, crushed

df gf

1 / In a bowl, mix together the salmon, mayonnaise, onions, pepper, dill, eggs, chia seeds and salt. Use your hands to shape the mixture into 8 round patties and set aside.

2 / Meanwhile, make the garlic aïoli. In a small bowl, mix together the avocado oil, mustard, lemon juice and crushed garlic.

3 / Gently heat the olive oil in a frying pan (skillet) over a low–medium heat, and fry the patties for 3–4 minutes on each side, or until they are golden.

4 / Serve with the garlic aïoli.

tips

I use chia seeds rather than flour in this recipe to bind the mixture, as the chia seeds contain less starch and are more nutritious. But, if you don't have any chia seeds to hand, you can use almond or a different flour to bind.

Try using avocado mayonnaise instead of regular in the fish cakes – it is made from avocado oil and high in oleic acid (an omega-9 fatty acid), which is thought to be anti-inflammatory with immunity-supporting properties.

If you want to spice it up, add 3 tsp curry paste to the fish cake mixture.

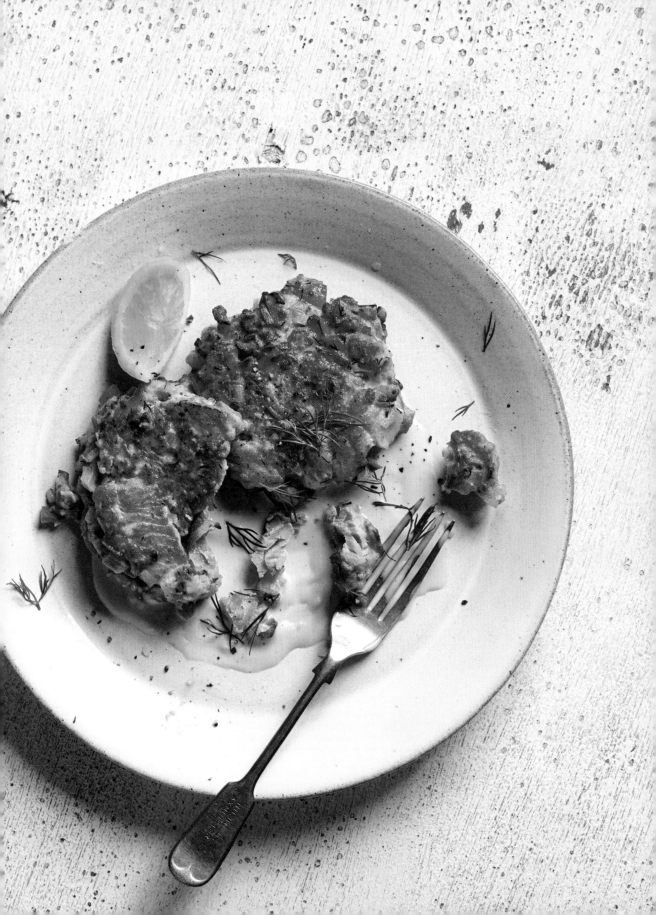

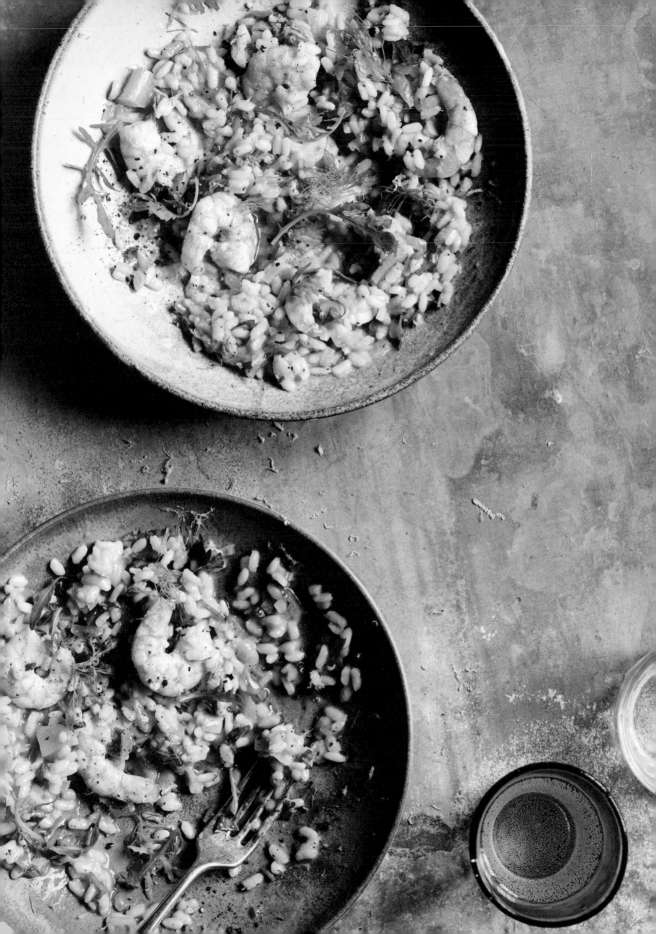

prawn and fennel risotto

I love this risotto, as the flavours work perfectly together. Prawns (shrimp) are a good source of selenium, one of the most effective antioxidants at maintaining healthy cells. They also contain high levels of zinc, which is important for supporting a healthy immune system. Fennel is a great prebiotic food source, which helps to fuel our beneficial gut bacteria.

Serves 4

2 Tbsp olive oil

1 onion, finely chopped

2 garlic cloves, finely chopped

1 small fennel bulb, cored and finely chopped

280g (10oz/1½ cups) risotto rice

1 litre (34fl oz/4 cups) hot vegetable stock (bouillon)

320g (11½oz) raw king prawns (jumbo shrimp)

zest and juice of ½ lemon

100g (3½oz) rocket (arugula), roughly chopped

sea salt (kosher salt) and freshly ground black pepper

df gf

1 / Gently heat the olive oil in a large saucepan over a low heat. Add the onion, garlic and fennel and cook for 8–10 minutes until softened. Add the rice and cook for 1–2 minutes, stirring constantly, until toasted. Add a ladleful of hot stock and stir until absorbed. Gradually add the remaining stock a ladleful at a time until it has all been absorbed and the rice is almost cooked (20–25 minutes). Add the prawns and lemon zest and juice, then season with a pinch of sea salt and some freshly ground black pepper. Cook for a further 4–5 minutes until the prawns are pink.

2 / Remove from the heat, stir in the rocket, and season to taste with extra black pepper.

options

For a vegan version, omit the prawns and add an extra onion and double the amount of rocket (you may also wish to use a whole lemon).

tips

Spice it up by adding 2 tsp ground cumin and 1 tsp ground turmeric.

pea and lemon risotto

This is such an easy and quick risotto made with green peas, which are high in fibre. They are also a great source of plant-based protein and contain multiple vitamins and minerals.

Serves 4

350g (12oz/1¾ cups) risotto rice

1.7 litres (60fl oz/7½ cups) hot vegetable stock (bouillon)

100g (3½oz/¾ cup) frozen peas

50g (2oz/¾ cup) grated Parmesan

zest and juice of 1 lemon

freshly ground black pepper

To serve:
green salad

gf

1 / Toast the rice in a large dry pan over a medium heat, stirring constantly for 1–2 minutes. Add a ladleful of hot stock and stir until absorbed, then reduce the heat. Gradually add the remaining stock a ladleful at a time until it has all been absorbed and the rice is almost cooked (20–25 minutes). Stir in the peas and cook for a further 3–5 minutes.

2 / Remove the pan from the heat, add the Parmesan and lemon juice, stirring well. Season with freshly ground black pepper, sprinkle over the lemon zest and serve with a large green salad.

options
For a vegan version, replace the Parmesan with a vegan cheese.

anchovy and tomato risotto

Anchovies are high in protein, iron, calcium, zinc and omega-3 fatty acids, which have been shown to decrease inflammation.

Serves 4

1 Tbsp extra-virgin olive oil

2 small onions, finely chopped

8 anchovy fillets in oil, drained

2 garlic cloves, crushed

280g (10oz/1½ cups) risotto rice

1.5 litres (50fl oz/6 cups) low-salt vegetable stock (bouillon)

½ tsp paprika

2 x 400g (14oz) cans chopped tomatoes

handful of basil leaves, chopped

80g (3oz/1 cup) Parmesan shavings

freshly ground black pepper

gf

1 / Gently heat the oil in a saucepan over a low heat. Add the onions and cook for 3 minutes, then add the anchovies and garlic, and cook for a further 3 minutes, stirring frequently. Add the risotto rice, stirring to coat it in the oil, and sauté for 2–3 minutes until it becomes translucent. Gradually add the stock a ladleful at a time, ensuring all the stock is absorbed before adding more and stirring continuously (20–25 minutes). Stir in the paprika and tomatoes and cook until the tomatoes are tender.

2 / Remove from the heat, season with freshly ground black pepper and scatter over the chopped basil and Parmesan shavings.

tips
Canned anchovies are high in sodium, so if you are following a low-sodium diet, you may wish to substitute the anchovies for tuna (opt for canned tuna in spring water rather than brine). I also recommend using low-salt stock for this reason.

This dish is versatile and can be made with quinoa in place of the risotto rice.

artichoke and mushroom spelt

Spelt is a type of grain that is an excellent source of fibre and also contains some vitamins and minerals. It is strongly related to wheat and has a similar nutritional profile. However, comparisons have demonstrated it to be slightly higher in protein and zinc.

Serves 4

200g (7oz/1¼ cups) dried spelt

300g (10½oz) artichokes preserved in oil, drained and halved

3 carrots, grated

20 cherry tomatoes, halved

large handful of olives

3 Tbsp olive oil

150g (5½oz) mushrooms, sliced

2 garlic cloves, crushed

freshly ground black pepper

To serve:
mixed green salad

Homemade Vinaigrette
(see page 198)

df vg

1 / Bring a large saucepan of water to the boil and cook the spelt according to the packet instructions.

2 / Drain the spelt and transfer to a mixing bowl, then add the artichokes, carrots, cherry tomatoes, olives and 2 tablespoons of the olive oil. Stir to coat the veggies with the oil and season with black pepper.

3 / In a separate pan, gently heat the remaining 1 tablespoon of olive oil over a low heat. Add the mushrooms and garlic and fry until the mushrooms are softened, then stir into the spelt mixture.

4 / Serve with a mixed green salad and vinaigrette.

options
For a gluten-free option, replace the spelt with quinoa.

tips
You can use any type of olives in this dish – I tend to use a mixture of black and green olives.

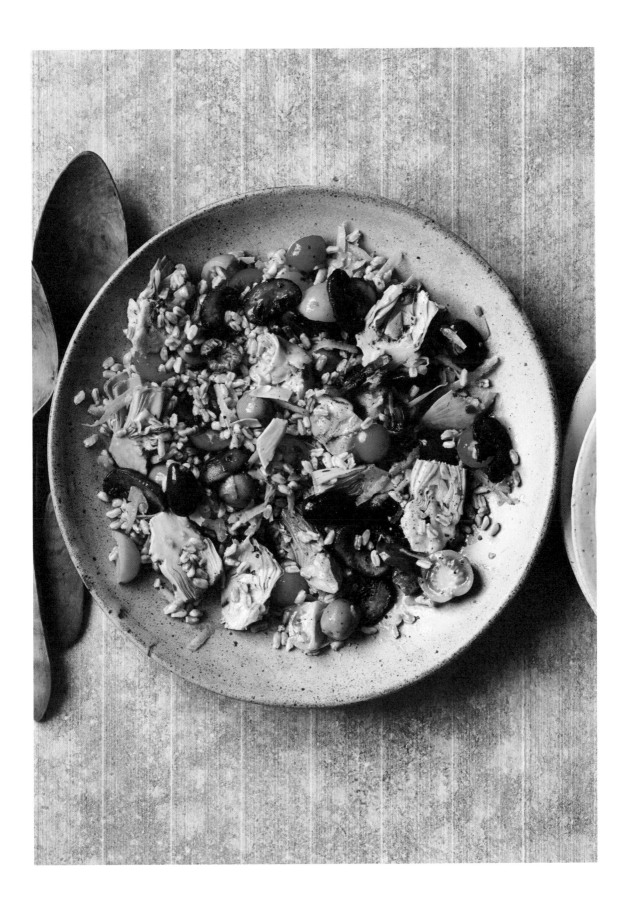

spicy lamb meatballs

This is a tasty, protein-packed recipe, which you can also enjoy the following day as a lunchbox lunch. These meatballs are delicious seasoned with rosemary, which is a member of the Lamiaceae mint family, along with other herbs such as basil, thyme, oregano and lavender. The rosemary not only tastes delicious, but also provides iron, calcium and vitamin B6.

Serves 4

500g (1lb 2oz) minced (ground) lamb

small handful of flat-leaf parsley, finely chopped

1 egg

2 garlic cloves, crushed

1 tsp dried chilli (red pepper) flakes

large bunch of rosemary, finely chopped

freshly ground black pepper

For the sauce:
2 Tbsp olive oil

2 onions, finely chopped

2 x 400g (14oz) cans chopped tomatoes

1 tsp hot smoked paprika

To serve:
320g (11½oz) wholegrain pasta, cooked

1 / Preheat the oven to 180°C (350°F/gas 4).

2 / Combine the lamb, parsley, egg, garlic, chilli flakes and rosemary in a bowl and mix well. Use your hands to shape the mixture into small balls, then place them on a baking sheet, ensuring they are spaced apart. Pop in the oven for 18–20 minutes, or until they are cooked through.

3 / Meanwhile, make the sauce. Gently heat the olive oil in a saucepan over a low heat. Add the onions and sweat for 5 minutes until softened. Add the tomatoes and paprika, and simmer for 12 minutes.

4 / Remove the meatballs from the oven, add them to the sauce and cook for a further 8 minutes.

5 / Season to taste with freshly ground black pepper, and serve with pasta.

options
For a gluten-free version, serve with rice pasta.

df

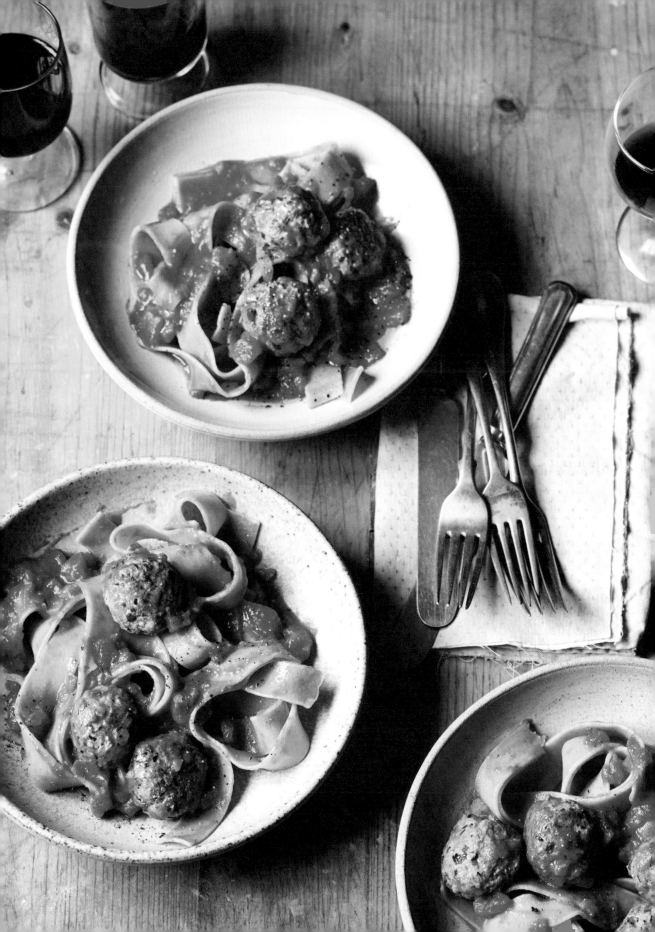

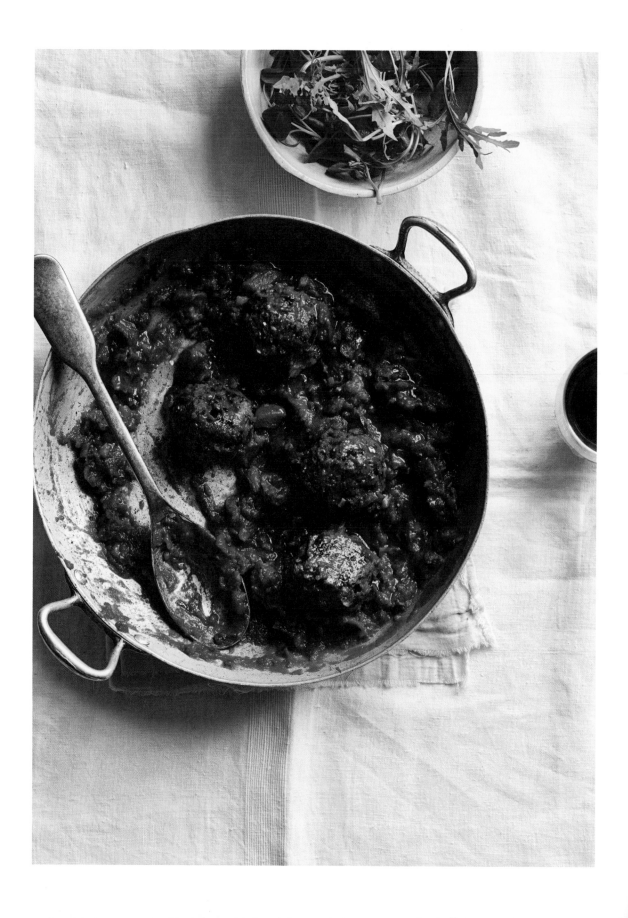

paprika and cayenne pepper 'meatballs'

This is a plant-based dish packed with fibre and antioxidants. Aubergines are the main veggie used in this dish and they are very nutrient dense, not only being an excellent source of fibre, but also a good source of vitamins B1, B6 and the minerals potassium, copper, magnesium and manganese. Aubergines are rich in antioxidants, particularly nasunin, which is found in the skin and gives the aubergine its purple colour.

Serves 4

For the 'meatballs':
1 Tbsp olive oil

1 red onion, finely chopped

2 garlic cloves, finely chopped

500g (1lb 2oz) aubergine (eggplant), diced

1 tsp paprika

1 tsp cayenne pepper

70g (2½oz/scant 1 cup) rolled (old-fashioned) oats

1 Tbsp flax seeds (linseeds)

For the tomato sauce:
2 Tbsp olive oil

2 red onions, finely chopped

1 garlic clove, finely chopped

1 tsp paprika

1 tsp cayenne pepper

2 x 400g (14oz) cans chopped tomatoes

freshly ground black pepper

To serve:
mixed salad or sautéed kale

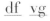

1/ Preheat the oven to 180°C (350°F/gas 4).

2/ First, make the 'meatballs'. Gently heat the olive oil in a saucepan over a low heat. Add the onion, garlic, aubergine, paprika and cayenne pepper, and cook for 5–8 minutes.

3/ Place the oats and flax seeds into a food processor and blitz to resemble a breadcrumb texture, then transfer to a bowl and set aside.

4/ Meanwhile, transfer the onion and aubergine mixture to the food processor and blitz for 1–2 minutes.

5/ Combine the onion and aubergine mixture with the oat mixture, then roll into 8 balls and place on a baking sheet, spaced slightly apart. Bake for 20–25 minutes until golden and cooked through.

6/ Meanwhile, make the tomato sauce. Gently heat the olive oil in a separate saucepan over a low–medium heat. Add the onions and garlic, and cook for 5 minutes. Add the paprika, cayenne pepper and tomatoes, then reduce the heat and simmer for 15 minutes, stirring occasionally.

7/ Remove the 'meatballs' from the oven, then add them to the sauce and cook for a further 3–5 minutes.

8/ Season with freshly ground black pepper, and serve with a mixed salad or on a bed of sautéed kale.

options
For a gluten-free version, use gluten-free oats instead of regular rolled oats.

tips
If you think the 'meatball' mixture could do with firming up before rolling into balls, then pop it in the fridge for 10–15 minutes first.

This tastes great with a little extra spice, so try adding a red chilli to the tomato sauce.

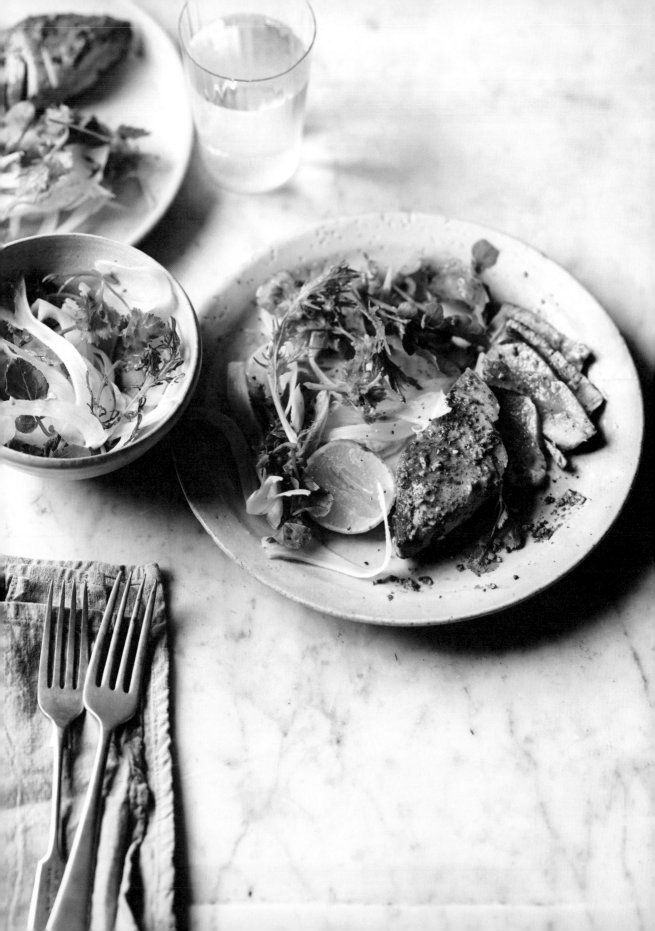

tangy tuna steaks

Tuna is an excellent source of protein and omega-3 fatty acids, and is also rich in manganese, zinc, vitamin C and selenium, which help to support the immune system.

Serves 4

2 garlic cloves

½ tsp chilli powder

½ tsp ground cumin

½ tsp paprika

small bunch of fresh coriander (cilantro)

juice of ½ lemon

160ml (5½fl oz/scant ¾ cup) olive oil

4 tuna steaks

sea salt (kosher salt) and freshly ground black pepper

To serve:
1 lime, cut into wedges

mixed salad

Homemade Vinaigrette
(see page 198)

 df gf

1 / Put the garlic, chilli powder, cumin, paprika, coriander and lemon juice into a blender or food processor, and blitz to a smooth purée. With the motor running, gradually add the olive oil until combined, then set aside.

2 / Arrange the tuna steaks in a non-reactive dish and cover with three-quarters of the dressing. Pop into the fridge for 30 minutes to marinate.

3 / When ready to cook, heat a frying pan (skillet) over a medium heat, add the tuna steaks and season with a pinch of sea salt and some freshly ground black pepper. Depending on the thickness of the steaks, cook for 2–4 minutes on each side, turning once.

4 / Serve with the remaining dressing poured over, with lime wedges and a large mixed salad dressed with vinaigrette.

tips

You can leave the tuna to marinate for longer than 30 minutes, if you like.

If you prefer your tuna well done, cook for an extra 2 minutes on each side.

This dish also tastes great served with a tomato and bean salad.

fruity lamb tagine

This is a very nutritious tagine that is ultra-easy to make! It is loaded with spices that taste fantastic and also benefit health. Cumin is naturally rich in iron and research suggests that it may play a role in weight loss, too. One study of 88 overweight women found that those who ate a little less than a teaspoon of cumin a day while on a low-calorie diet lost more body fat and weight than those on the same diet who didn't add cumin to their diet.

Serves 4

400g (14oz) stewing lamb, diced

3 Tbsp olive oil

2 red onions, diced

1 yellow (bell) pepper, deseeded and diced

1 red (bell) pepper, deseeded and diced

2 garlic cloves, finely chopped

1 tsp ground cumin

1 tsp ground ginger

1 tsp ground cinnamon

100g (3½oz/¾ cup) dried apricots, quartered

500ml (18fl oz/2 cups) chicken stock (bouillon), or more as needed

1 x 400g (14oz) can chopped tomatoes

1 small butternut squash, peeled, deseeded and cut into 1cm (½in) cubes

freshly ground black pepper

To serve:
handful of pine nuts, toasted

100ml (3½fl oz/scant ½ cup) organic Greek yoghurt

gf

1 / Preheat the oven to 180°C (350°F/gas 4).

2 / Combine all the ingredients in a large casserole dish and cover with the lid. Cook in the oven for 1½ hours, removing the lid and stirring after 1 hour. Check occasionally and add more stock during cooking, if required.

3 / Remove from the oven and season to taste with freshly ground pepper. Serve, sprinkled with the toasted pine nuts, with a dollop of Greek yoghurt.

options
For a vegan option, replace the lamb with the same weight of dried or canned lentils, use vegetable stock instead of chicken stock and serve with coconut or soy yoghurt.

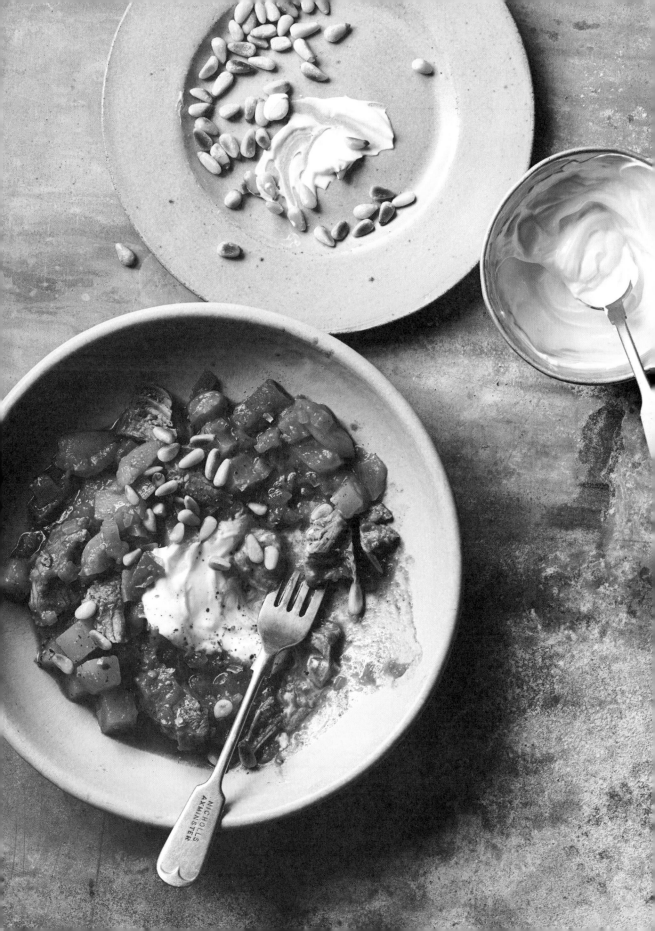

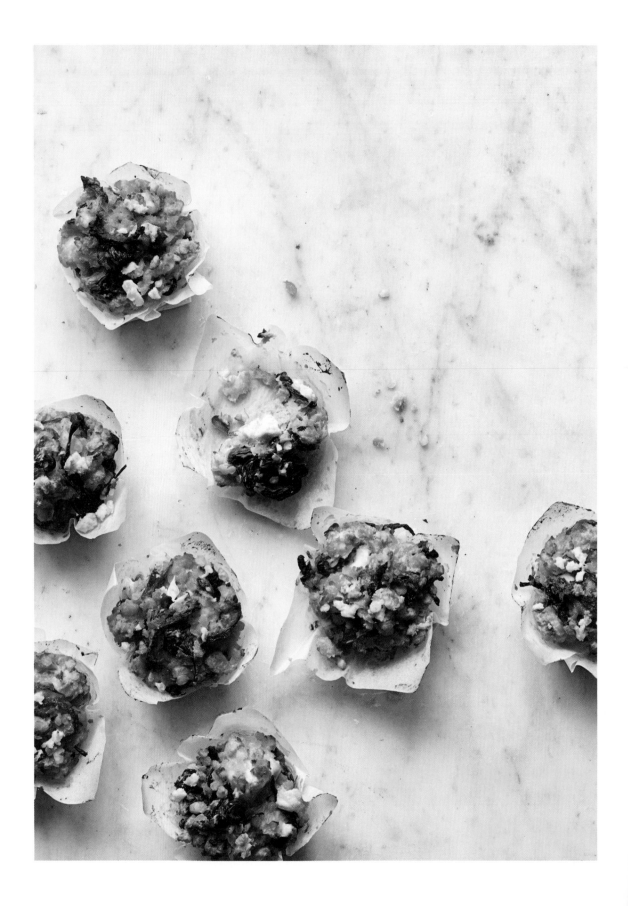

red lentil and rosemary patties

Red lentils are rich in vitamins A, B6 and folate. Rosemary is an ultra-fragrant herb that is rich in antioxidants, which prevent cell damage. Research has suggested that one of rosemary's compounds – 1,8-cineole – may even boost brain activity.

Serves 4

1 Tbsp olive oil, plus extra for greasing

300g (10½oz/scant 1¾ cups) dried red lentils

1 red onion, sliced

1 Tbsp balsamic vinegar

100g (3½oz) baby spinach

1 egg, beaten,

50g (2oz/⅓ cup) rice flour

100g (3½oz) feta, crumbled

1 tsp dried or finely chopped fresh rosemary

1 / Preheat the oven to 180°C (350°F/gas 4). Lightly grease an 8-hole muffin tin (pan) with a little olive oil (or see Tip).

2 / Put the lentils into a large pan with 500ml (18fl oz/2 cups) water and bring to the boil, then reduce the heat and simmer for 15 minutes until the water is absorbed.

3 / Gently heat the olive oil in a saucepan over a low heat. Add the onion and balsamic vinegar and allow the vinegar to evaporate and caramelize. Add the baby spinach and stir until wilted.

4 / Combine the cooked lentils with the onion and spinach mixture, egg, rice flour and feta. Divide the mixture between the 8 holes of the muffin tin, and sprinkle over the rosemary.

5 / Bake for 20 minutes until golden.

options
For a vegan or dairy-free option, replace the egg with an egg substitute such as 1 Tbsp apple sauce or 1 Tbsp chia seeds, and the feta with vegan cheese, such as hemp-seed-crumble cheese or a sprinkling of nutritional yeast.

tips
If you don't have a non-stick muffin tin, you can line each hole with a square of baking paper instead.

These taste delicious served with Sweet Potato Wedges (page 192) and Crunchy Coleslaw (page 193).

broccoli lemon chicken with cashews

Chicken breast is high in protein, low in fat, and is also a great source of iron, zinc, selenium and B vitamins. I use cashew nuts in this dish, and not only do they taste great, but they are a powerhouse of vitamins, minerals and other beneficial nutrients.

Serves 4

2 Tbsp olive oil

3 small skinless chicken breasts, sliced into strips

250g (9oz) Tenderstem broccoli, stems halved

2 garlic cloves, finely chopped

200ml (7fl oz/scant 1 cup) chicken stock (bouillon), or more as needed

1 Tbsp honey

80g (3oz/½ cup) cashew nuts

grated zest and juice of 1 lemon

To serve:
quinoa or Cauliflower Rice
(see page 192)

df gf

1 / Gently heat the olive oil in a wok over a low–medium heat, add the chicken strips and stir-fry for 8–10 minutes until golden and cooked through. Remove to a plate and set aside.

2 / Add the broccoli and garlic to the wok and stir-fry for 3–4 minutes. Combine the stock and honey, then pour into the wok and stir until thickened (you may need to increase the heat slightly to thicken it). Return the chicken to the wok, add the cashew nuts, lemon zest and juice, and heat through. Add more stock, if required, to achieve the desired consistency.

3 / Serve with quinoa or cauliflower rice.

options
For a vegan option, replace the chicken with 300g (10½oz) tofu.

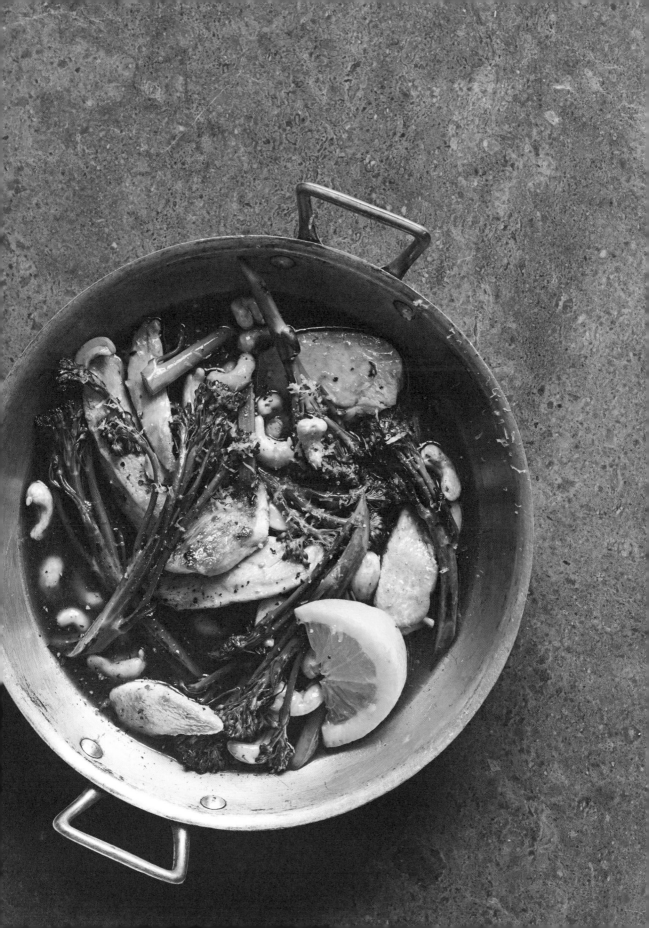

mediterranean lamb steaks

Not only is lamb a rich source of high-quality protein, but it is also an excellent source of many vitamins and minerals, including iron, zinc and vitamin B12.

Serves 4

2 Tbsp olive oil

2 red onions, chopped

4 lamb steaks

2 tsp rice flour or chickpea (gram) flour

2 garlic cloves, chopped

1 fresh rosemary sprig

small bunch of fresh oregano

750ml (25fl oz/3¼ cups) lamb or vegetable stock (bouillon)

400g (14oz/2 cups) chopped tomatoes, fresh or canned

freshly ground black pepper

To serve:
Mediterranean Roasted Vegetables (see page 191)

df gf

1 / Preheat the oven to 180°C (350°F/gas 4).

2 / Heat 1 tablespoon of the oil in a sauté pan over a low–medium heat. Add the onions and gently brown for 5 minutes, stirring frequently. Remove to a plate and set aside.

3 / Coat the lamb steaks in the flour and add the remaining tablespoon of oil to the pan. Put the steaks in the pan and cook for 4 minutes on each side, turning once. Return the onions to the pan and add the garlic, rosemary and oregano. Pour in the stock, stir well and slowly bring to the boil. Add the tomatoes, season with freshly ground black pepper and cook for a further 2 minutes, stirring well.

4 / Transfer to an ovenproof dish and pop in the oven for 30 minutes. After 30 minutes, cover the dish with foil and cook for a further 15 minutes.

5 / Season to taste with freshly ground black pepper and serve with Mediterranean roasted vegetables.

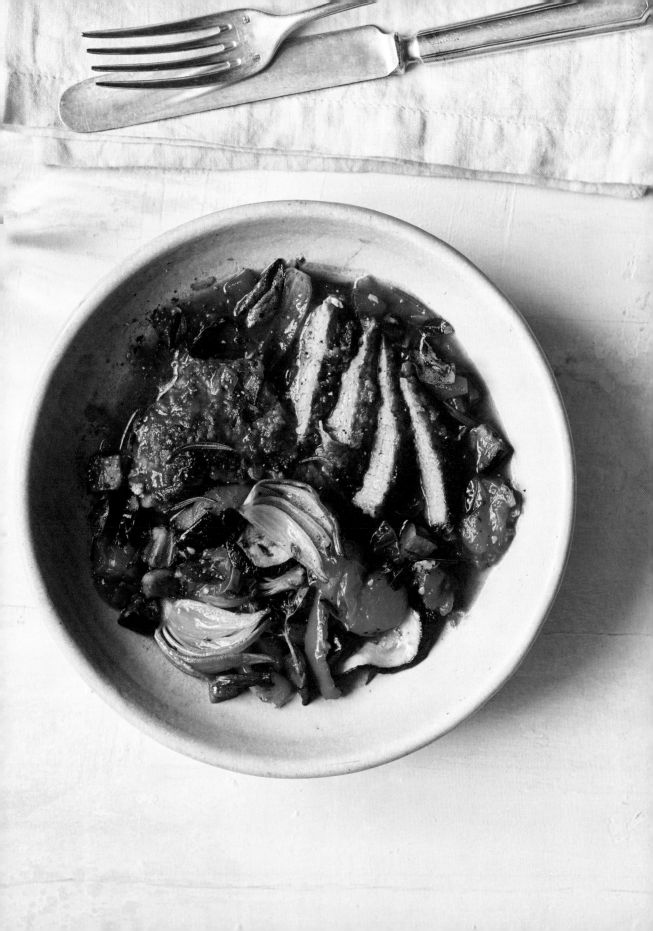

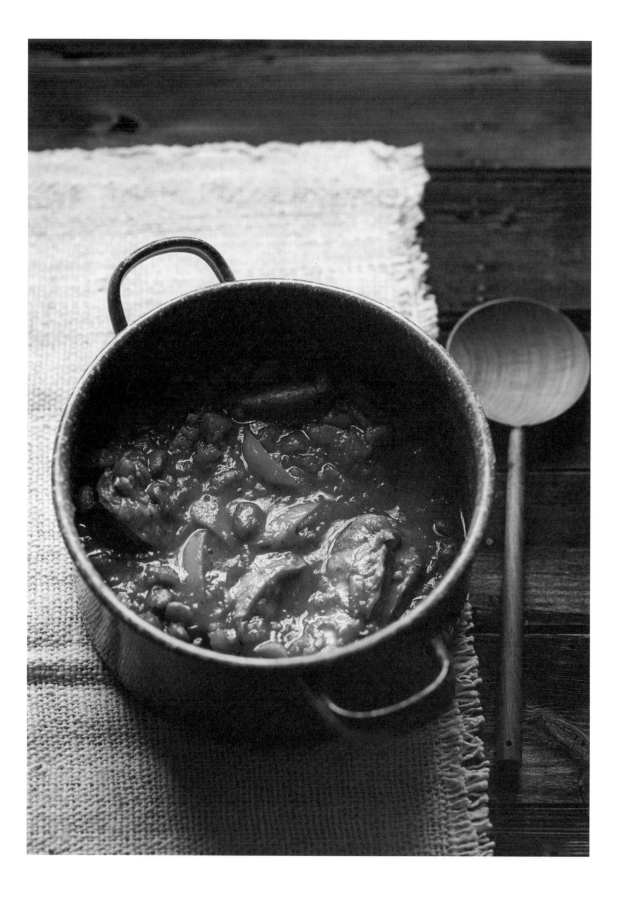

hearty chicken casserole

I make this casserole with chicken breast, which is high in protein but low in fat. Chicken is a great source of vital nutrients, including iron, zinc, selenium and B vitamins. If you prefer the darker thigh meat, do feel free to use it in place of the breast meat.

Serves 4

1 Tbsp olive oil

4 small skinless chicken breasts

2 red onions, chopped

3 garlic cloves, crushed

1 yellow (bell) pepper, deseeded and chopped

1 red (bell) pepper, deseeded and chopped

1 Tbsp tomato purée (paste)

1 x 200g (7oz) can borlotti (cranberry) beans, drained and rinsed

2 x 400g (14oz) cans chopped tomatoes

250ml (8fl oz/1 cup) chicken stock (bouillon), or more as needed

2 tsp dried marjoram

freshly ground black pepper

df gf

1 / Heat the oil in a sauté pan over a low–medium heat. Add the chicken breasts, then increase the heat and cook for about 8 minutes on each side, or until golden.

2 / Add the onions, garlic and peppers, and cook for a further 3 minutes.

3 / Add the tomato purée, beans, tomatoes, chicken stock and marjoram and stir well. Season with freshly ground black pepper and bring to the boil, then cover, reduce the heat and simmer gently for 40–45 minutes. Add more stock if it's looking dry during cooking.

4 / Season to taste with freshly ground black pepper before serving.

options
For a vegan option, replace the chicken breasts with 400g (14oz/1¾ cups) pinto beans or chickpeas (garbanzo beans), and use vegetable stock in place of the chicken stock.

puy lentils with smoked tofu

I make this dish with Puy lentils, which come from Le Puy in France. They are similar in colour to green lentils, but are about a third of the size, with a peppery taste. They are packed with B vitamins and the minerals magnesium, potassium and zinc.

Serves 4

1 Tbsp olive oil

1 onion, finely sliced

2 carrots, finely diced

1 courgette (zucchini), finely chopped

1 red or yellow (bell) pepper, deseeded and finely diced

200g (7oz) smoked tofu, finely chopped

1 tsp smoked paprika

2 Tbsp balsamic vinegar

500g (1lb 2 oz/generous 3 cups) cooked Puy (French) lentils

juice of ½ lemon

handful of fresh dill, chopped

freshly ground black pepper

<u>df</u> <u>gf</u> <u>vg</u>

1 / Gently heat the olive oil in a saucepan over a low heat. Add the onion, carrots, courgette, pepper, tofu and smoked paprika, and cook for 8–10 minutes until the vegetables are tender, stirring frequently. Add the balsamic vinegar and stir for a further 2 minutes until the vinegar starts to sizzle.

2 / Put the lentils into a large bowl, then add the tofu and vegetable mixture and mix well. Squeeze over the lemon juice and stir through, then scatter over the dill and season with freshly ground black pepper.

tips

You can use any vegetables you have to hand in this dish – it is ultra-versatile.

If you are short on time, use canned or vacuum-packed cooked Puy lentils.

Try crumbled feta on top if you aren't dairy-free or vegan – it's delicious!

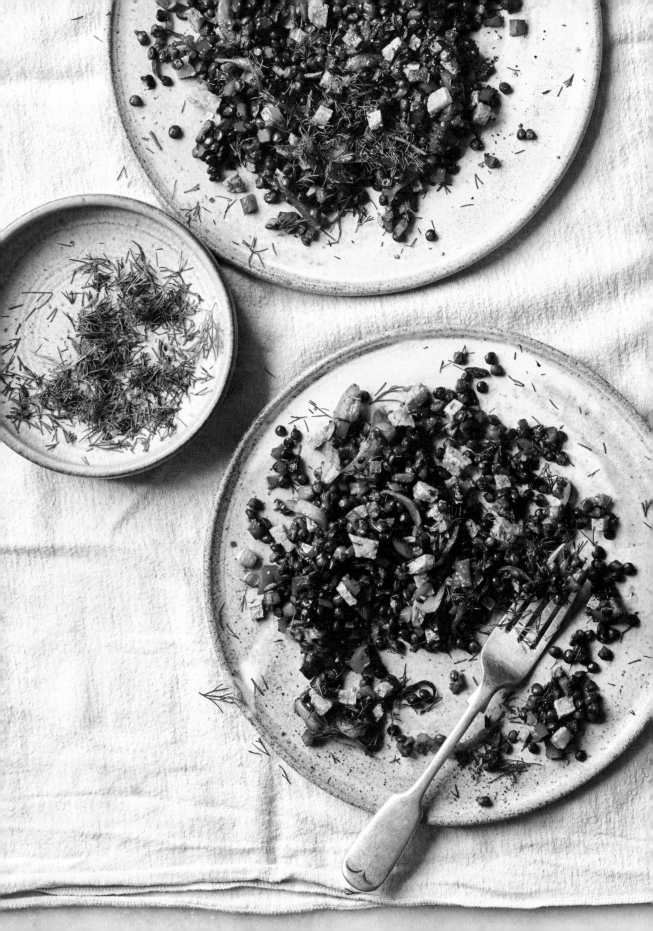

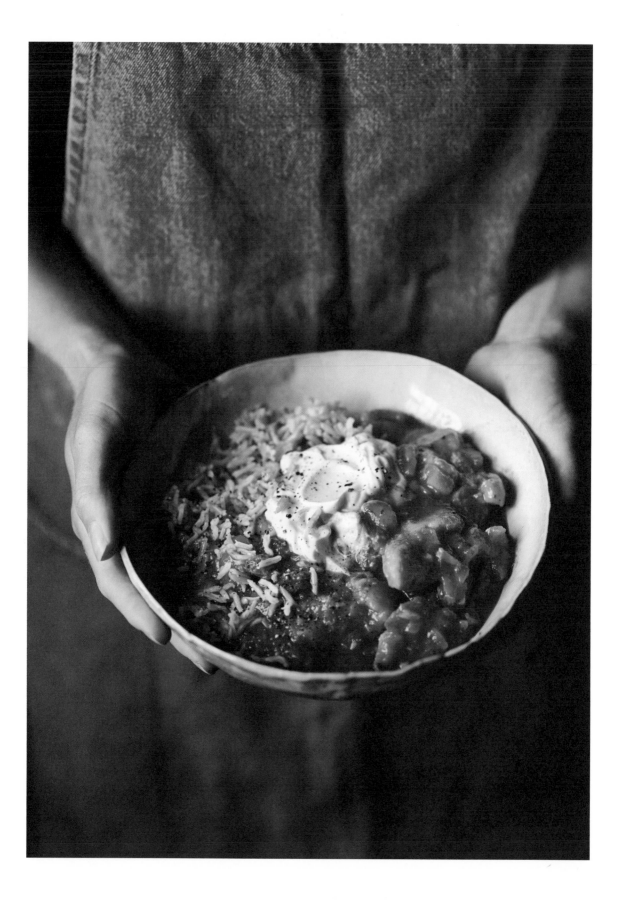

chicken banana korma

Children love this korma – it is a great way to introduce spiced foods into younger family members' diets. It is much healthier than a standard takeaway korma, too!

Serves 4

2 Tbsp olive oil

500g (1lb 2oz) skinless chicken breast, diced

1 large onion, finely chopped

2 garlic cloves, crushed

2 Tbsp korma curry paste

500ml (18fl oz/2 cups) chicken stock (bouillon), or more as needed

80g (3oz/⅔ cup) dried apricots, chopped

handful of sultanas (golden raisins)

1 banana, sliced

freshly ground black pepper

To serve:
80ml (2½fl oz/¾ cup) organic Greek yoghurt

250g (9oz/1¼ cups) brown rice
or 1 x recipe quantity Cauliflower Rice (see page 192)

1 / Gently heat the olive oil in a saucepan over a low heat. Add the chicken, onion and garlic and cook for 5 minutes, stirring frequently. Increase the heat, then add the curry paste, stock, apricots and sultanas. Stir well and bring to the boil, then reduce the heat and simmer for 30–35 minutes, adding more stock, if required. Add the sliced banana and cook for a further 5 minutes.

2 / Season to taste with freshly ground black pepper and serve topped with Greek yoghurt, with brown rice or cauliflower rice on the side.

options

For a vegan version, replace the chicken with 350g (12oz) tofu, the chicken stock with vegetable stock, and the Greek yoghurt with coconut yoghurt.

For a dairy-free version, replace the Greek yoghurt with coconut yoghurt.

chilli and coconut salmon

Salmon is rich in astaxanthin, a powerful antioxidant that gives salmon its lovely pink colour. Astaxanthin has also been shown to reduce the risk of heart disease, improve blood flow, and decrease oxidative stress. In addition, several studies have reported that this potent antioxidant may lower inflammation and pain associated with the autoimmune disease rheumatoid arthritis.

Serves 4

1 Tbsp coconut oil (see Tip)

2 onions, finely chopped

2 garlic cloves, crushed

3cm (1in) piece of fresh root ginger, grated

1 red chilli, finely sliced

1 tsp ground turmeric

300ml (10fl oz/1¼ cups) fish stock (bouillon), or more as needed

300ml (10fl oz/1¼ cups) coconut cream

4 Tbsp fresh lemongrass

4 wild salmon fillets

2 Tbsp fish sauce

handful of fresh dill, chopped

sea salt (kosher salt) and freshly ground black pepper

To serve:
Cauliflower Rice (see page 192)

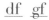

1 / Gently heat the coconut oil in a saucepan with a lid over a low heat. Add the onions, garlic, ginger, chilli and turmeric, and cook for 5 minutes, then increase the heat, add the fish stock, coconut cream and lemongrass and bring to the boil. Add the salmon, cover the pan, then reduce the heat and simmer for 8–10 minutes until the fish is cooked through, adding a little more stock, if required. Remove the salmon to a bowl and set aside.

2 / Meanwhile, prepare the cauliflower rice according to the instructions on page 192.

3 / Bring the sauce back to the boil and cook for a further 5 minutes, then remove from the heat and stir in the fish sauce. Season with a pinch of salt and some freshly ground black pepper.

4 / Pour the sauce into bowls, add the salmon, scatter over the fresh dill, and serve with the cauliflower rice.

tips

If you don't have fresh lemongrass to hand, use the zest of 1–2 lemons instead.

To spice it up even more, use 2 red chillies.

Make your own Coconut Oil to use in this recipe (see page 200).

Farmed salmon contains up to three times more saturated fat than wild salmon, and wild salmon is higher in minerals, such as iron, zinc and potassium, so do opt for wild over farmed if possible.

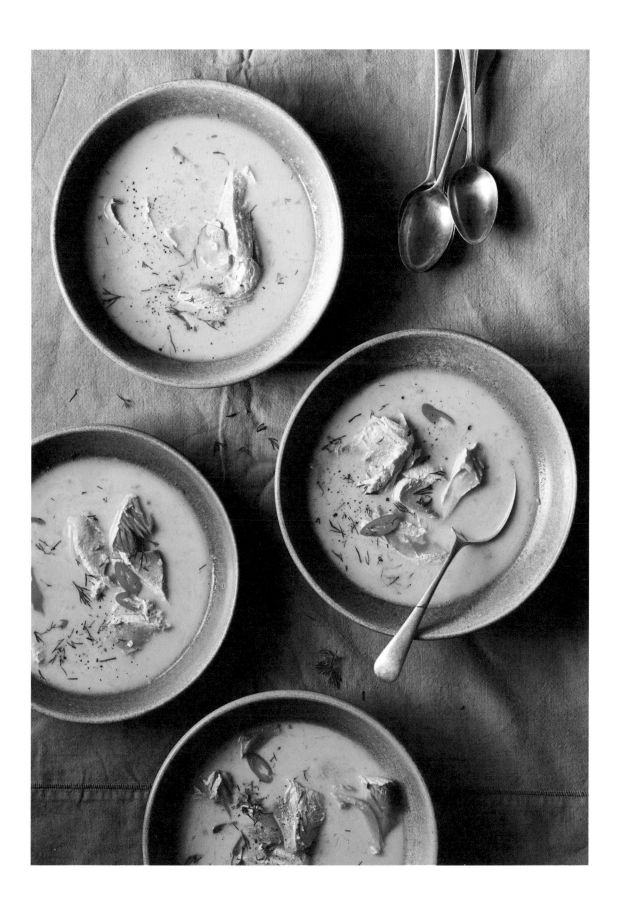

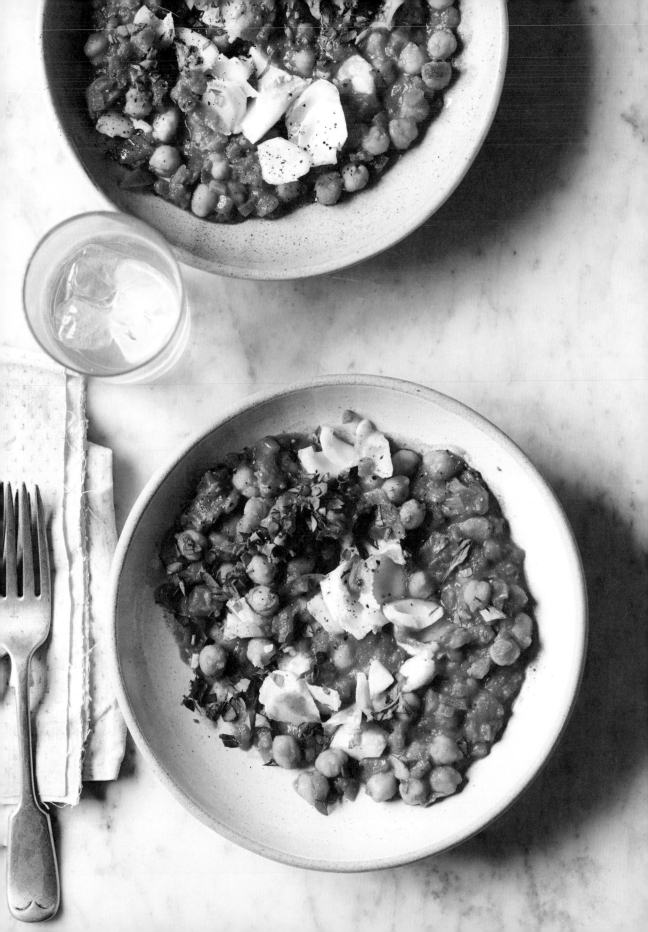

moroccan fish stew

There is nothing like a bowl of warm stew to lift the spirits, and the cinnamon and cumin are wonderful additions to this dish. Cinnamon is a spice that has been prized for its medicinal properties for thousands of years. It contains large amounts of powerful polyphenol antioxidants, which have anti-inflammatory effects that may help decrease your risk of disease. Cinnamon is also high in cinnamaldehyde, which is thought to be responsible for most of its health benefits.

Serves 4

2 Tbsp olive oil

1 red onion, chopped

2 garlic cloves, crushed

2 tsp ground cumin

2 tsp ground turmeric

1 cinnamon stick

500g (1lb 2oz) haddock, cut into chunks

1 x 400g (14oz) can chopped tomatoes

1 x 400g (14oz) can chickpeas (garbanzo beans), drained

1 red chilli, thinly sliced

handful of flat-leaf parsley, finely chopped

freshly ground black pepper

df gf

1 / Gently heat the olive oil in a saucepan over a low heat. Add the onion and sweat for 5 minutes until softened, then add the garlic, cumin, turmeric and cinnamon stick and cook for 2 minutes, stirring occasionally. Add the fish, tomatoes, chickpeas and chilli along with 250ml (8fl oz/1 cup) water. Bring to the boil and simmer for 6–8 minutes, or until the fish is cooked through.

2 / Season to taste with freshly ground black pepper, remove the cinnamon stick and sprinkle with the parsley to serve.

options
For a vegan option, replace the fish with mixed beans.

tips
You can use any white fish in this recipe – pollock or ling are great substitutes.

butter bean stew

Butter beans, also known as lima beans, are a superb source of fibre, iron and B vitamins. They also provide manganese, zinc, magnesium, potassium, phosphorus and valuable antioxidants. They pack a powerful protein punch, but since they are considered an incomplete protein, because they don't offer all of the amino acids required by your body, I always serve this dish with rice to make this bean stew a complete protein dish.

Serves 4

2 Tbsp olive oil

2 red onions, diced

3 celery sticks, finely chopped

2 carrots, sliced

2 x 400g (14oz) cans butter (lima) beans, drained

800g (1lb 12oz) ripe tomatoes, skinned and chopped

3 garlic cloves, crushed

1 tsp ground cinnamon

1 tsp paprika

1 Tbsp sundried tomato paste

handful of flat-leaf parsley, chopped

freshly ground black pepper

To serve:
cooked rice or lentils

df gf vg

1 / Preheat the oven to 180°C (350°F/gas 4).

2 / Gently heat the olive oil in a large saucepan over a low heat. Add the onions, celery and carrots, and cook for 5 minutes, or until soft and tender. Add the butter beans, tomatoes, garlic, cinnamon, paprika and sundried tomato paste, and cook for a further 5 minutes. Transfer to a casserole dish, cover and cook in the oven for 40–45 minutes, checking occasionally and adding a little water if it starts to look dry.

3 / Remove from the oven, sprinkle with the parsley and season with freshly ground black pepper. Serve with your chosen accompaniment.

tips
If you are short on time, use canned tomatoes instead of fresh.

Spice it up with 1–2 tsp chilli powder.

Make sure you serve with rice or lentils, as this will make this wonderful dish of beans a meal that has complete protein.

tuna and bean patties

I use borlotti (cranberry) beans in this recipe and they work really well with the tuna. Borlotti beans are an inexpensive source of protein, low in fat, while being very high in fibre. They are also a good source of copper, manganese, potassium and magnesium, which are all minerals that are essential to health.

Serves 4

1 x 400g (14oz) can borlotti (cranberry) beans

1 egg white

1 garlic clove

small handful of flat-leaf parsley

1 red onion, quartered

400g (14oz) tuna, fresh and finely chopped, or canned

freshly ground black pepper

To serve:
mixed salad

Crunchy Coleslaw (see page 193)

df gf

1 / Preheat the oven to 180°C (350°F/gas 4).

2 / Put the beans, egg white, garlic, parsley and onion into a food processor and blitz to a purée, then transfer to a large bowl. Mix in the tuna until well combined and season with freshly ground black pepper.

3 / Use your hands to shape the mixture into 8 patties and place on a baking sheet. Bake in the oven for 12–15 minutes, or until golden, turning halfway through cooking.

4 / Serve with a mixed salad and coleslaw.

options

For a vegan option, replace the tuna with cannellini beans and use an egg substitute or chia seeds instead of the egg white.

If you prefer a less nutty taste, use cannellini beans instead of borlotti beans.

tips

You can use any beans you have to hand for this recipe – kidney beans, pinto beans or black beans.

If you want to spice it up, add 1 Tbsp Thai red curry paste to the recipe.

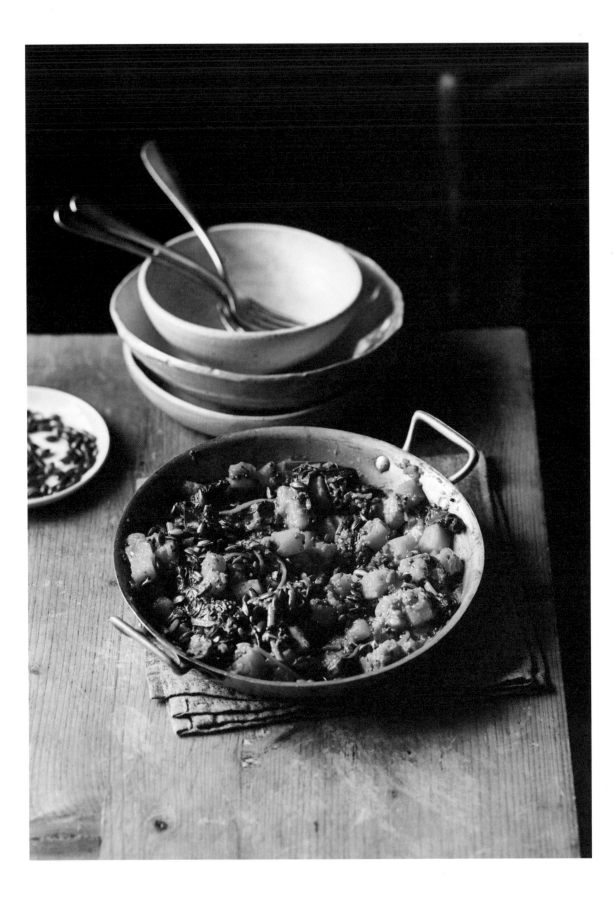

pumpkin and spinach curry

Pumpkin and spinach are high in fibre and potassium, both of which support digestion. This dish is delicious with the fresh ginger, which is one of my favourite spices to use in cooking. Ginger is high in gingerol, a substance with powerful anti-inflammatory and antioxidant properties, which benefit health.

Serves 4

1 Tbsp olive oil

1 onion, chopped

2 garlic cloves, finely chopped

3cm (1in) piece of fresh root ginger, grated

1 tsp ground cumin

1 tsp ground turmeric

1 tsp ground coriander

1 medium pumpkin, peeled and diced

1 Tbsp mustard seeds

150ml (5fl oz/⅔ cup) passata (strained tomatoes)

200ml (7fl oz/scant 1 cup) vegetable stock (bouillon), or more as needed

250g (9oz) spinach

handful of pumpkin seeds, toasted

freshly ground black pepper

df gf vg

1 / Gently heat the olive oil in a large saucepan over a low heat. Add the onion, garlic and ginger and sweat for 5 minutes until softened. Add the cumin, turmeric and ground coriander and cook for 2 minutes, then add the pumpkin, mustard seeds, passata, vegetable stock and a grinding of black pepper. Simmer for 20 minutes, adding more water or stock, if required.

2 / Stir in the spinach and cook for a final 2 minutes. Season to taste with black pepper and scatter with the toasted pumpkin seeds.

tips

If you don't have pumpkin to hand, use butternut squash instead.

This can be served with Cauliflower Rice (see page 192) or wholegrain rice.

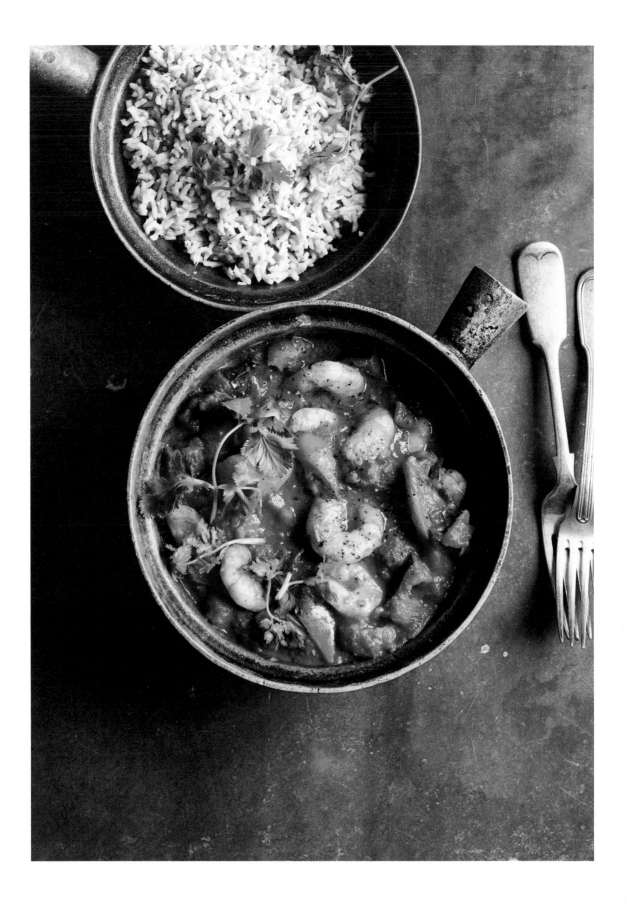

king prawn jalfrezi

Prawns (shrimp) are high in protein and an excellent source of selenium, one of the most effective antioxidants at maintaining healthy cells. They also provide high levels of vitamin B12, vitamin E and the mineral phosphorus. They are a good source of zinc, which plays a vital role in supporting the immune system. In addition, this dish is packed with phytochemicals from all the wonderful yellow, green, red and purple vegetables included.

Serves 4

2 Tbsp olive oil

2 onions, chopped

2 garlic cloves, chopped

2cm (¾in) piece of fresh root ginger, finely chopped

1 tsp ground coriander

1 tsp ground cumin

1 tsp ground turmeric

½ tsp dried chilli (red pepper) flakes

2 x 400g (14oz) cans chopped tomatoes

1 small aubergine (eggplant), chopped

1 green (bell) pepper, deseeded and chopped

1 yellow (bell) pepper, deseeded and chopped

250g (9oz) cooked king prawns (jumbo shrimp)

small bunch of fresh coriander (cilantro), chopped

freshly ground black pepper

To serve:
280g (10oz/scant 1½ cups) wholegrain brown rice, cooked, or 1 x recipe quantity Cauliflower Rice (see page 192)

df gf

1 / Gently heat the olive oil in a large saucepan over a low heat. Add the onions, garlic and ginger, and cook for 5 minutes until softened. Add the coriander, cumin, turmeric, chilli flakes and a twist of black pepper, then sir in the tomatoes, aubergine and peppers, cover and simmer for 10–12 minutes. Stir in the prawns and cook for a further 3 minutes.

2 / Season to taste with black pepper, scatter with the fresh coriander, and serve with wholegrain brown rice or cauliflower rice.

options
For a vegan version, replace the prawns with chickpeas (garbanzo beans).

tips
Homemade raita (see page 119) is delicious with this dish.

spiced kedgeree

Kedgeree is a dish high in protein, healthy fats, vitamins and minerals. I make this with brown rice, as it is nutrient dense and provides you with all the fibre and vitamins (namely B vitamins) that you need. A delicious blend of spices, which provide antioxidant and anti-inflammatory properties, make this dish a really healthy and delicious supper.

Serves 4

2 Tbsp olive oil

2 small onions, finely chopped

1 red chilli, deseeded and chopped

3 Tbsp curry powder

1 tsp mustard seeds

1 tsp cayenne pepper

1 tsp ground turmeric

300g (10½oz) smoked haddock fillet

handful of fresh coriander (cilantro), chopped

4 eggs, hard-boiled and quartered

freshly ground black pepper

For the spiced rice:
2 Tbsp olive oil

1 large onion, finely chopped

1 tsp ground coriander

1 tsp medium curry powder

280g (10oz/scant 1½ cups) easy-cook long-grain brown rice, rinsed

df gf

1 / Start with the spiced rice. Gently heat the olive oil in a large saucepan over a low heat. Add the onion and sweat for 5 minutes until softened, then add the ground coriander and curry powder and cook for 3 minutes. Add the rice along with 600ml (20fl oz/ 2½ cups) water and bring to the boil, then reduce the heat, cover and simmer for 12 minutes. Remove from the heat and leave to stand for 15 minutes, covered.

2 / Gently heat the olive oil in a separate saucepan over a low heat. Add the onions and chilli and cook for 5 minutes, then add the curry powder, mustard seeds, cayenne pepper and turmeric, and cook for a further 2 minutes. Mix in the cooked rice, haddock and fresh coriander and gently heat through for 2–3 minutes.

3 / Season with freshly ground black pepper, and serve with the quartered eggs on top.

options
For a vegan option, replace the fish and eggs with a 400g (14oz) can chickpeas (garbanzo beans) and add extra vegetables.

tips
Make sure you leave the rice covered until the end of cooking, as it will be cooked perfectly then.

This is such a versatile dish – you can use any vegetables you have to hand. I have used carrots, red (bell) pepper and peas before and it tasted delicious!

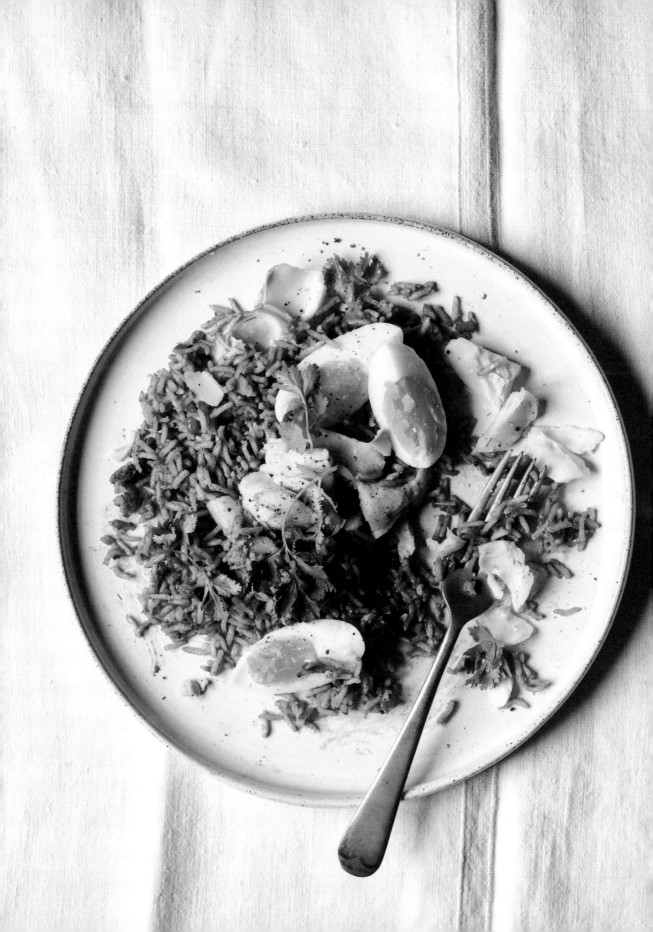

kimchi fried rice

This recipe is a great way to include kimchi in your diet, as well as use up leftover rice. You can buy the kimchi or make your own (see page 196).

Serves 4

3 Tbsp olive oil, plus 1 tsp (optional)

2 garlic cloves, finely sliced

3cm (1in) piece of fresh root ginger, grated

300g (10½oz) Tenderstem broccoli, chopped

1 large white onion, thinly sliced

4 spring onions (scallions), finely sliced

100g (3½oz) kimchi (store-bought or see page 196)

320g (11½oz/generous 1½ cups) wholegrain rice, cooked

3 carrots, cut into ribbons using a vegetable peeler

4 eggs

2 limes: 1 juiced; 1 cut into wedges

large handful of fresh coriander (cilantro), chopped

freshly ground black pepper

df gf

1 / Gently heat the 3 tablespoons of oil in a large pan over a low heat. Add the garlic, ginger, broccoli, white onion and 3 of the spring onions, and cook for 6 minutes until softened. Add the kimchi and cook for 2–3 minutes, then stir in the rice and the carrots and heat through.

2 / Meanwhile, add the 1 teaspoon of oil, if needed, to a frying pan (skillet) set over a low–medium heat. Crack in the eggs and cook to your preference.

3 / Squeeze the lime juice over the rice and divide it among individual bowls. Place the eggs on top of the rice, scatter with the last spring onion, sprinkle over the coriander, and season to taste with freshly ground black pepper. Serve with the lime wedges.

options
For a vegan version, use nori strips instead of the egg for topping.

tips
You can replace the rice in this dish with quinoa or millet.

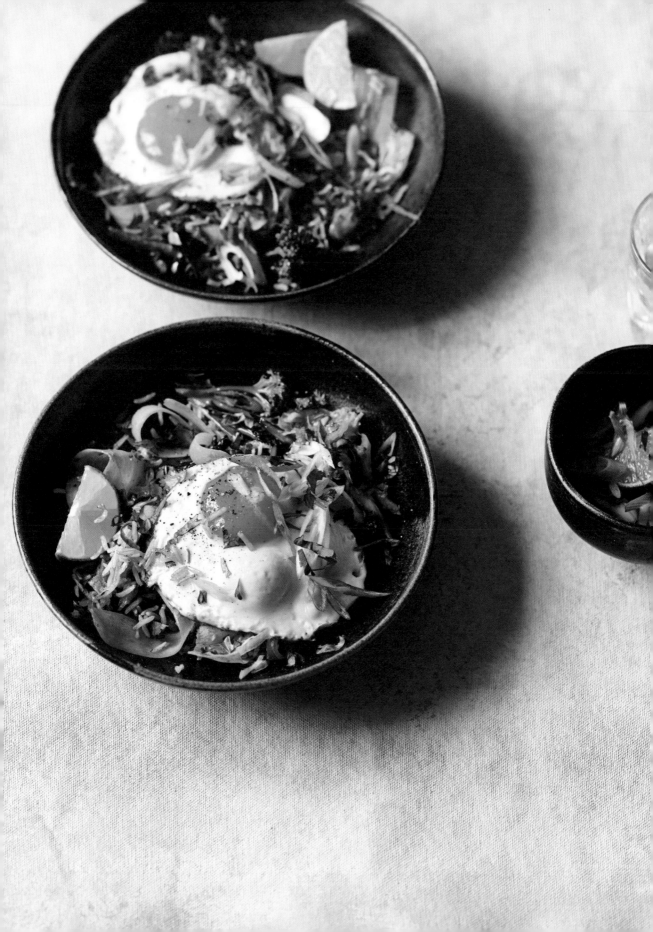

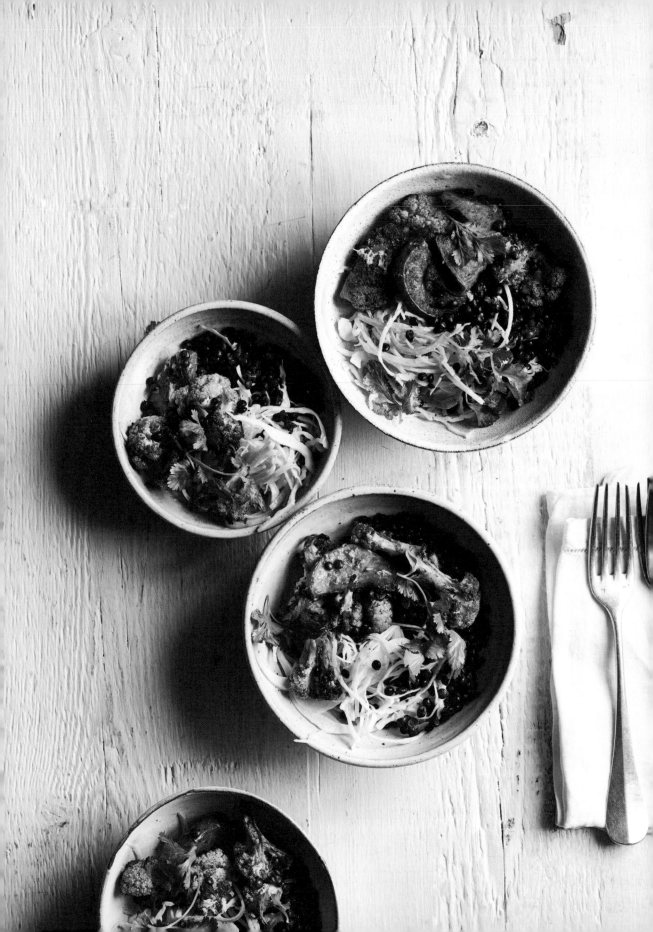

cauliflower, lentil and sweet potato bowl

This is a fabulously tasty plant-based dish, and each bowl contains four of your five-a-day! It keeps really well in the fridge, so you can cook a batch and have it as a lunchbox lunch the next day.

Serves 4

1 cauliflower, cut into florets

1 large sweet potato, cut into bite-size chunks

2 garlic cloves, sliced

1 Tbsp garam masala

4 Tbsp olive oil

250g (9oz/1¼ cups) Puy (French) lentils

1 tsp Dijon mustard

3cm (1in) piece of fresh root ginger, grated

juice of 1 lemon

handful of fresh coriander (cilantro), chopped

freshly ground black pepper

To serve:
Crunchy Coleslaw (see page 193)

df gf vg

1 / Preheat the oven to 180°C (350°F/gas 4).

2 / In a large bowl, mix together the cauliflower, sweet potato, garlic and garam masala with 2 tablespoons of the olive oil. Arrange the veggies in a roasting tin (pan) and roast in the oven for 35 minutes.

3 / Meanwhile, put the lentils into a saucepan along with 500ml (18fl oz/ 2 cups) water and bring to the boil. Reduce the heat and simmer for 25 minutes, or until the lentils are cooked. Drain and set aside.

4 / In another large bowl, mix the remaining 2 tablespoons of olive oil with the mustard, ginger and half of the lemon juice, then stir in the cooked lentils.

5 / Divide the lentils among 4 serving bowls, then top with the roasted cauliflower and sweet potato. Scatter over the fresh coriander and squeeze over the remaining lemon juice.

6 / Season to taste with freshly ground pepper and serve with coleslaw.

pesto courgetti

Courgettes (zucchini) contain very few calories and have a high water content. They provide immune-system-supporting vitamin C, and significant levels of potassium, which is key to controlling blood pressure. A great way to get courgettes into your diet is as courgetti, using it to replace pasta. I make this courgetti with pesto and it is simply delicious.

Serves 4

2 tsp olive oil

3 garlic cloves, finely chopped

6 courgettes (zucchini), spiralized (see Tip)

80g (3oz/generous ½ cup) pine nuts

handful of basil leaves

handful of mint leaves

80g (3oz/1¼ cups) grated Parmesan

drizzle of extra-virgin olive oil

freshly ground black pepper

1 / Gently heat the olive oil in a saucepan over a low heat. Add the garlic and cook until softened, then add the courgetti and cook, stirring, until all the water in the courgettes has evaporated.

2 / Meanwhile, toast the pine nuts in a separate dry pan over a low heat until golden, stirring continuously.

3 / Remove the courgetti from the heat and tip into a large serving bowl. Add the basil, mint, toasted pine nuts and Parmesan and mix well. Drizzle with extra-virgin olive oil, season to taste with freshly ground black pepper and serve.

options
For a vegan or dairy-free option, replace the Parmesan with ground almonds and nutritional yeast flakes.

tips
Don't worry if you don't have a spiralizer, you can also use a julienne peeler to peel the courgette into lengthways strips.

Add 4 big handfuls of frozen peas and you can serve this as a main dish.

mediterranean roasted vegetables

This is a brilliant way of meeting your five-a-day veggie goal in one meal. This dish contains vegetables in all the different colours, which makes this super-high in antioxidants.

Serves 4

6 Tbsp olive oil

4 garlic cloves, crushed

1 aubergine (eggplant), diced

2 small courgettes (zucchini), sliced

1 large red onion, sliced

2 red (bell) peppers, deseeded and sliced

1 yellow (bell) pepper, deseeded and sliced

20 cherry tomatoes

1 rosemary sprig, chopped

1 thyme sprig, chopped

pinch of sea salt (kosher salt)

freshly ground black pepper

df gf vg

1 / Preheat the oven to 160°C (325°F/gas 3).

2 / In a small bowl, mix together the oil and garlic.

3 / Put the aubergine, courgettes, onion, peppers and tomatoes into a large roasting tin (pan), mix together well and arrange in a single layer. Drizzle with the oil and garlic mixture and sprinkle with the rosemary, thyme and sea salt. Roast in the oven for 45–50 minutes until tender.

4 / Season to taste with freshly ground black pepper.

tips
This is such a versatile dish, you can use any combination of vegetables you wish.

When roasting the veggies, do spread them out well so they don't go soggy.

If you are short on time, cheat by using bags of ready-chopped vegetables.

Adding some feta to this can transform it into a great lunchbox lunch for the next day.

sweet potato wedges

Sweet potatoes are high in fibre and antioxidants, which help protect our bodies from free radical damage and chronic disease, encourage the growth of beneficial gut bacteria and promote a healthy gut. These wedges can accompany literally any main dish or even be enjoyed on their own as a light supper with Homemade Mayo (see page 198).

Serves 4

4 medium-sized sweet potatoes, peeled and cut into wedges

4 Tbsp olive oil

1 tsp paprika

1 tsp cayenne pepper

½ tsp sea salt (kosher salt)

df gf vg

1 / Preheat the oven to 200°C (400°F/gas 6).

2 / Spread the sweet potato wedges over a baking sheet and sprinkle with the olive oil, paprika, cayenne pepper and sea salt. Pop in the oven for 20 minutes.

3 / Remove from the oven and gently shake the tray to turn the wedges, then return to the oven and cook for a further 20 minutes until they are golden and crispy.

cauliflower rice

This is a brilliant low-carb alternative to rice and it contains more nutrients. It is also a great prebiotic food source and packed with fibre.

Serves 4

1 cauliflower

4 tsp tahini

1 Tbsp olive oil

1 tsp ground turmeric

½ tsp sea salt (kosher salt)

handful of fresh coriander (cilantro), finely chopped

freshly ground black pepper

df gf vg

1 / Preheat the oven to 200°C (400°F/gas 6).

2 / Blitz the cauliflower in a blender or food processor until it resembles grains.

3 / In a large bowl, combine the cauliflower with the tahini, olive oil, turmeric and sea salt.

4 / Spread the mixture out in a thin layer over a baking sheet and bake in the oven for 10–12 minutes.

5 / Just before serving, season to taste with freshly ground black pepper and stir in the finely chopped fresh coriander.

tips
You can transform this into a main dish by frying 120g (4½oz) cooked chicken pieces with 3 Tbsp cooked peas, then mixing this into the cauliflower rice.

crunchy coleslaw

Cabbage contains many different antioxidants that have been shown to reduce chronic inflammation. In fact, research has shown that eating more cruciferous vegetables reduces certain blood markers of inflammation. It is rich in vitamin K and vitamin C, and while both green and red cabbage are excellent sources of vitamin C, red cabbage contains about 30 per cent more than white cabbage. It is also one of my favourite prebiotic food sources, providing fuel for the beneficial bacteria in our guts.

Serves 4

½ white cabbage, finely sliced

½ red cabbage, finely sliced

2 carrots, grated

4 spring onions (scallions), trimmed and chopped

2 tsp avocado oil

1 tsp wholegrain mustard

2 Tbsp avocado mayonnaise

2 Tbsp natural (plain) yoghurt

2 Tbsp sunflower seeds, toasted

sea salt (kosher salt) and freshly ground black pepper

gf

1 / Combine the cabbage, carrots and spring onions in a large bowl and stir in the avocado oil, mustard, mayonnaise and yoghurt. Season with a pinch of sea salt and some freshly ground black pepper and scatter over the sunflower seeds.

options
For a vegan option, omit the yoghurt and replace with an extra 2 Tbsp avocado mayonnaise (do check the label, as some avocado mayonnaise products contain egg).

For a dairy-free option, omit the yoghurt and replace with an extra 2 Tbsp avocado mayonnaise.

tips
Don't worry if you don't have avocado mayo to hand, just use regular mayonnaise.

I love to jazz this up by using purple cabbage, which not only gives it a bright look, but is rich in anthocyanin – a pigment with powerful antioxidant properties.

pak choi with oyster sauce

Pak choi, also known as bok choy, contains vitamins C, E and beta-carotene. These nutrients have powerful antioxidant properties that help protect cells against damage by free radicals. Pak choi is also a great prebiotic food source, which fuels the beneficial gut bacteria.

Serves 4

2 Tbsp olive oil

2 garlic cloves, roughly chopped

4 heads pak choi (bok choy), leaves separated

1 Tbsp soy sauce

2 Tbsp oyster sauce

1 red chilli, deseeded and finely sliced (optional)

df

1 / Heat the olive oil in a wok over a low heat. Add the garlic and cook for 2 minutes, then add the pak choi, stirring until it wilts. Add 3 tablespoons of water along with the soy sauce and oyster sauce and simmer for 2–3 minutes.

2 / Serve, scattered with the chilli, if using.

options
For a vegan option, replace the oyster sauce with a vegan stir-fry sauce of your choice.

For a gluten-free option, replace the soy sauce with tamari (and check the oyster sauce is gluten-free).

tips
Pak choi can be substituted with other Chinese vegetables, such as choi sum, kai lan, or even broccoli.

ratatouille

High in fibre and antioxidants, this vegetable side dish can even be made as a main dish. It is also delicious with feta crumbled on top. For a vegan and dairy-free alternative, sprinkle with nutritional yeast.

Serves 4

1 Tbsp olive oil

2 courgettes (zucchini), chopped

1 yellow (bell) pepper, deseeded and chopped

1 orange (bell) pepper, deseeded and chopped

2 red onions, cut into wedges

2 garlic cloves, chopped

handful of fresh basil, chopped

5 ripe tomatoes, chopped

1 x 400g (14oz) can chopped tomatoes

1 Tbsp balsamic vinegar

sea salt (kosher salt) and freshly ground black pepper

df gf vg

1 / Gently heat the olive oil in a sauté pan over a low–medium heat. Add the courgettes and peppers, and cook for 5–7 minutes until softened..Remove to a large bowl and set aside.

2 / Meanwhile, add the onions, garlic and basil to the same pan and cook for 8–10 minutes. Return the courgettes and peppers to the pan, add the tomatoes and balsamic vinegar, then cover and simmer on a low heat for 30 minutes.

3 / Season with a pinch of sea salt and some freshly ground black pepper to taste.

tips
Opt for whatever vegetables are in season.

Spice it up by adding 1 tsp chilli powder.

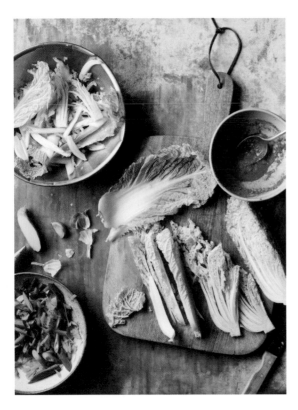

kimchi

This wonderful Korean dish is said to be one of the secrets to the Koreans' longevity!

Makes 2 x 500ml (18fl oz/1 pint) jars

1 Chinese cabbage, or other cabbage of choice, cut into 2–3cm (¾–1in) strips

1 Tbsp sea salt (kosher salt)

3 garlic cloves, crushed

3cm (1in) piece of fresh root ginger, grated

2 Tbsp fish sauce

1 tsp chilli powder

1 tsp paprika

3 Tbsp rice vinegar

3 spring onions (scallions), diced

3 carrots, grated

df gf

tips

The flavour improves the longer it is left – I tend to leave it for 2 weeks so the flavour can really develop.

Kimchi is delicious eaten with eggs. I often add some to an omelette for a super-quick supper.

1 / Put the cabbage into a large bowl, add the sea salt and massage it into the cabbage for 5 minutes. Set aside for 1 hour.

2 / Meanwhile, in a separate bowl combine the garlic, ginger, fish sauce, chilli powder, paprika and rice vinegar.

3 / Drain the cabbage and rinse several times under cold running water to remove the excess salt. Dry thoroughly and place the cabbage back in a large bowl, along with the spring onions and carrots. Add the garlic mixture and toss through.

4 / Pack the mixture into two 500ml (18fl oz/1 pint) jars, pushing it well down and leaving a small space at the top of each jar. Put the lids on and leave to ferment at room temperature. Check on it every day or so and release any gas that may have built up as it is fermenting.

5 / After 3 days, taste it. If you prefer a more acidic taste, leave for another couple of days. Once it is ready, transfer it to the fridge, where it will keep for up to 2 weeks.

sauerkraut

Sauerkraut is packed with probiotic bacteria and one of the easiest fermented foods to make.

Makes 2 x 500ml (18fl oz/ 1 pint) jars

1kg (2lb 3oz) white cabbage, thinly shredded

4 tsp sea salt (kosher salt)

½ tsp peppercorns

½ tsp caraway seeds

1 / Put the shredded cabbage into a large clean bowl and add the salt, massaging it into the cabbage for 5 minutes. Leave for 3–5 minutes, then massage the cabbage again for a further 5 minutes. Mix in the peppercorns and caraway seeds.

2 / Pack the mixture into two 500ml (18fl oz/1 pint) jars, leaving a small space at the top of each to allow the cabbage mixture to fizz up. Push the cabbage well down so it is submerged in its juices, cover with the lids and leave in a dark place at room temperature for at least 5 days.

3 / Check on it every day or so and release any gas that may have built up as it is fermenting. If any yeasts form, just remove and discard. After 5 days, it will be ready to enjoy and it will keep in the fridge for up to 6 months.

tips
During the first five days, it is really important to keep it at an even room temperature: too warm and the sauerkraut may ferment too quickly or even become mouldy; too cold and it will take longer.

If your sauerkraut becomes too dry, you can top it up by adding 30ml (2 Tbsp) cool, filtered water, adding more as and when required. Use filtered water, as chlorine inhibits bacteria, which is the exact reason it is added to drinking water. You can de-chlorinate your tap water by boiling it with the lid of the kettle open so that the chlorine can escape.

I have made beetroot (beet) sauerkraut in the past, and it is delicious. Just add 400g (14oz) grated beetroot to the cabbage – give it a go!

homemade mayo

Making your own mayonnaise takes some patience, but it is so worth it, as it can accompany so many dishes. It keeps really well in the fridge, too

Makes 500ml (18fl oz/2 cups)

2 egg yolks

1 Tbsp Dijon mustard

500ml (18fl oz/2 cups) groundnut oil

1–2 Tbsp white wine vinegar

juice of ½ lemon

flaky sea salt (kosher salt) and freshly ground black pepper

df   gf

1 / Whisk the eggs in a bowl, then add the mustard and season with a pinch of sea salt and some freshly ground black pepper. Whisk together until completely combined.

2 / Slowly add a little of the oil, whisking constantly, then gradually add more of the oil, little by little, until the yolks and oil combine and start to thicken. Once you are happy the eggs and oil are coming together well, add more of the oil at a time. This takes patience, but if you add the oil too quickly the mayo will split and curdle. When you have added about half of the oil, whisk in 1 tablespoon of the vinegar, then continue to add the remaining oil gradually and whisking constantly.

3 / Season to taste, squeeze in the lemon juice, and add another tablespoon of vinegar, if required.

tips
Make sure all the ingredients are at room temperature before starting.

You can use any oil that you have to hand for making mayonnaise, or you can mix the oils up. Try making avocado mayonnaise by using avocado oil.

homemade vinaigrette

I always recommend that you make your own dressings, as homemade dressings such as this vinaigrette are healthier, being free of preservatives, added sugars and artificial flavourings.

Makes 200ml (7fl oz/scant 1 cup)

1 Tbsp raw apple cider vinegar

1 lemon: zest of the whole lemon and juice of ½

1 tsp Dijon mustard

200ml (7fl oz/scant 1 cup) extra-virgin olive oil

df   gf   vg

1 / Put all the ingredients, except the olive oil, into a bowl and blitz with a hand-held blender for a few seconds, then slowly pour in the oil.

tips
If you don't have raw apple cider vinegar or Dijon mustard to hand, a simple dressing of lemon juice, olive oil and ½ tsp honey will still taste delicious.

Add ¼ avocado, 1 tsp ground turmeric and 1 tsp honey to this base recipe and you have a great anti-inflammatory salad dressing.

pesto

Pesto is ultra-easy to make and very versatile. You can enjoy it as a dressing for salad or add to main dishes.

Makes about 150ml (5fl oz/⅔ cup)

50g (2oz/scant ½ cup) pine nuts

80g (3oz/2½ cups) fresh basil leaves

50g (2oz/¾ cup) grated Parmesan

150ml (5fl oz/⅔ cup) extra-virgin olive oil

2 garlic cloves, chopped

1 / Toast the pine nuts in a dry pan over a low heat until golden, shaking occasionally. Transfer to a blender or food processor, add the basil, Parmesan, olive oil and garlic and blitz until smooth.

2 / It will keep for up to 1 week in an airtight container in the fridge.

tips

I love adding a twist to traditional basil pesto by making kale pesto and coriander (cilantro) pesto! For the kale pesto, steam a small bunch of kale (stems removed) for 2–3 minutes, then add to the blender/food processor with the other ingredients as above. For coriander pesto, use 50g (2oz/2½ cups) fresh coriander (cilantro) leaves, add to the other ingredients as above and blitz in the blender.

nut butter

Who knew making your own nut butter would be so easy? It is ultra-versatile and can be enjoyed on a slice of wholegrain bread, or used in baking, in a salad dressing, or even to make your own sweet treats (see page 202).

Makes 1 x 250g (9oz) jar

250g (9oz/2 cups) almonds, hazelnuts or peanuts, skin on

1–2 tsp maple syrup or honey (optional)

df gf vg

1 / Preheat the oven to 190°C (375°F/gas 5).

2 / Arrange the nuts in a single layer on a baking sheet and cook in the oven for 10–12 minutes. Remove and set aside until cooled.

3 / Place the cooled nuts in a food processor or blender and blitz for about 10 minutes, stopping occasionally to scrape the mixture down from the sides. If you prefer a sweeter taste, add some maple syrup or honey and stir through.

4 / Pour into a jar and store in the fridge for up to 3 weeks.

coconut oil

For those of you who use coconut oil a lot, this recipe will be a blessing. The processing does require patience, but a good food processor or blender will deliver great results. Keep blitzing until the mixture is runny, and make sure to use a whole packet of coconut – any less than this will lack the volume needed to make it work.

Makes 1 x 500ml (18fl oz/1 pint) jar

1 x 500g (17½ oz) pack unsweetened shredded coconut

df gf vg

1 / Pour the shredded coconut into a blender and blitz for 2–3 minutes. If using a food processor, blitz for 12–15 minutes, or until the mixture is runny.

2 / Transfer the mixture to a jar or airtight container and store in the fridge. If making this in winter and your house is cool, you can store in the cupboard.

tips
If you are keeping this in the fridge, when you go to use it just scoop out a wedge and let it soften at room temperature before using it.

kefir

Kefir is a fermented milk drink and is similar to yoghurt. It is really easy to make, and is super-nourishing for both your gut and your immune system.

Serves 8

800ml (28fl oz/scant 3½ cups) organic full-fat (whole) milk

2 Tbsp kefir grains

You will also need 1 or 2 sterilized 1 litre (34fl oz/1 quart) glass jars or containers with a lid

gf

1 / Pour the milk into your sterilized container and add the kefir grains, stir and place the lid on. Keep it at room temperature (21–25°C/70–77°F) for 8–24 hours (if you live in a colder climate, you may need to leave for 30–48 hours).

2 / Taste to see if it is ready and to your liking. Once it is, strain it through a fine sieve (strainer) and pour into a sterilized airtight glass jar, bottle or container. Store in the fridge for up to 1 week.

tips
You can use the kefir grains again – just rinse them in filtered water, pat dry, place in an airtight container and pop them into the freezer. When you go to reuse the grains, put them in milk to defrost.

Try making fruity kefir – add a handful of ripe fresh berries or even mango to your kefir milk.

oat milk

This is a perfect alternative to milk if you have a lactose intolerance or dairy allergy, or if you are looking for a vegan alternative. Super-easy to make, it keeps in the fridge for 2–3 days. Shake well before use.

Makes about 750ml (25fl oz/3¼ cups)

100g (3½oz/1 cup) porridge oats (oatmeal/old-fashioned oats), gluten-free if necessary

pinch of sea salt flakes (kosher salt)

df gf vg

1 / Put the oats into a bowl and cover with water. Cover the bowl and leave for at least 4 hours or overnight, if possible.

2 / Drain the mixture in a sieve (strainer) and rinse under running water.

3 / Put the soaked oats into a blender or food processor along with 750ml (25fl oz/3¼ cups) water and add the pinch of salt. Blitz for a few minutes until smooth.

4 / Line a sieve (strainer) with a piece of muslin (cheesecloth), then place over a jug (pitcher) and pour in the liquid. Leave to strain for 60–75 minutes. To help speed up the process, scrape the bottom of the muslin occasionally to remove some of the residue. Once it has completely strained, if you prefer a thinner consistency, add a little water.

tips
When most of the liquid has gone through the sieve into the jug, gather the sides of the muslin together and squeeze tightly with both hands to extract the last of the milk.

I use the leftover oat pulp mixed with coffee grounds as a body scrub and it works a treat.

almond milk

Another great alternative to milk if you have a lactose intolerance or dairy allergy, or if you are looking for a vegan alternative. The process for making almond milk is similar to oat milk (see left) – it is super-easy and keeps in the fridge for 2–3 days. Shake well before use.

Makes about 750ml (25fl oz/3¼ cups)

150g almonds

df gf vg

1 / Put the almonds into a bowl and cover with water. Cover the bowl and leave for at least 4 hours or overnight, if possible.

2 / Drain the mixture in a sieve (strainer) and rinse under running water.

3 / Put the soaked nuts into a blender or food processor along with 750ml (25fl oz/3¼ cups) water and blitz for a few minutes until smooth.

4 / Line a sieve (strainer) with a piece of muslin (cheesecloth), then place over a jug (pitcher) and pour in the liquid. Leave to strain for 60–75 minutes. To help speed up the process, scrape the bottom of the muslin occasionally to remove some of the residue. Once it has completely strained, if you prefer a thinner consistency, add a little water.

tips
When most of the liquid has gone through the sieve into the jug, gather the sides of the muslin together and squeeze tightly with both hands to extract the last of the milk.

Use in porridge, smoothies and baked goods.

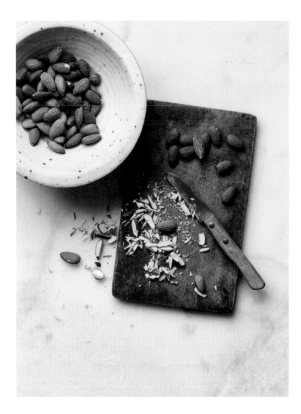

almond crunch

My absolute favourite recipe – it always satisfies a sugar craving without any white refined sugar and it can be made with just 2 teaspoons of maple syrup. Almonds are a source of protein, healthy fats, fibre, magnesium and vitamin E.

Makes 20 pieces

80g (3oz/⅓ cup) coconut oil (see Tip), melted

5 Tbsp almond butter

2 Tbsp desiccated (unsweetened dried shredded) coconut

2 tsp maple syrup

pinch of sea salt (kosher salt)

df gf vg

1 / Line a small baking dish with baking paper.

2 / In a bowl, mix the melted coconut oil, almond butter, coconut and maple syrup until well combined. Pour onto the baking paper and sprinkle with a pinch of sea salt.

3 / Place in the freezer for 15–20 minutes until firm to the touch.

4 / Remove from the freezer and cut into pieces.

tips

If you like this extra crunchy, use crunchy almond butter instead of smooth.

If you don't have almond butter to hand, you can use peanut butter or hazelnut butter.

If you are looking to make this for children, leave out the salt and use 4 tsp maple syrup instead. If you are trying to reduce your child's sugar intake, or your own, this is a brilliant chocolate and sweet (candy) substitute.

Keep in the fridge in an airtight container – this treat can last up to 4–5 days, if you can resist it for that long!

Make your own Coconut Oil to use in this recipe (see page 200).

chocolate avo mousse

Avocados are one of the most nutritious foods on the planet. They are packed with fibre, more soluble fibre than any other fruit in fact, and contain several vitamins, including the antioxidant vitamins C and E. They also provide the powerful antioxidants beta-carotene and lutein, which are extremely beneficial to our health.

Serves 4

2 ripe avocados, halved, stones removed and flesh scooped out

3 Tbsp unsweetened cocoa powder or raw cacao powder

2 Tbsp maple syrup, or more to taste

2 tsp vanilla bean paste or vanilla extract

1 / Put the avocado flesh into a blender or food processor, add the cocoa powder or raw cacao powder, maple syrup, vanilla bean paste and 1 tablespoon of water. Blitz until the mixture is smooth. Taste, and add more maple syrup, if required.

2 / Divide the mixture among 4 serving glasses or small bowls, and chill in the fridge for 3 hours before serving.

tips
If you like this even creamier with a hint of coconut, add 1 Tbsp coconut cream.

If you don't have vanilla bean paste or extract to hand, don't worry – it tastes just as good without.

Experiment – try a minty version by adding ¼ tsp mint extract. Alternatively, try fruity chocolate mousses, adding a handful of frozen raspberries or mango to the blender when you blitz. Children love a banana chocolate version – just add a small banana to the ingredients and blitz.

raspberry coconut chocolate

This is another of my favourite homemade chocolate recipes, packed with antioxidants from the raspberries and raw cacao powder. Raw cacao is one of the best food sources of magnesium, which is a mineral essential for energy production, brain health, supporting the nervous system, and for bone health. It is also a source of iron, as well as potassium, copper, zinc, manganese and selenium. In addition to this, raw cacao also contains a compound called phenylethylamine (PEA), which is believed to promote energy and boost mood. In fact, it is said to be one of the reasons why people like chocolate so much!

Makes 20 pieces

80g (3oz/⅓ cup) coconut oil (see Tip)

80g (3oz/⅓ cup) butter

2 Tbsp raw cacao or unsweetened cocoa powder

4 tsp maple syrup

80g (3oz/1 cup) frozen raspberries

60g (2½oz/¾ cup) desiccated (unsweetened dried shredded) coconut

gf

1 / Line a baking dish with baking paper.

2 / Melt the coconut oil and butter in a saucepan over a low heat. Stir in the raw cacao or cocoa powder and maple syrup, stirring well.

3 / Pour the chocolate mixture onto the baking paper and scatter over the raspberries and coconut. Place in the freezer for 25–30 minutes, until firm to the touch.

4 / Remove from the freezer and cut into pieces.

tips

This will keep for up to 4 days in an airtight container in the fridge.

Try experimenting by adding nuts and raisins instead of raspberries – this is great fun to do with children.

Make your own Coconut Oil to use in this recipe (see page 200).

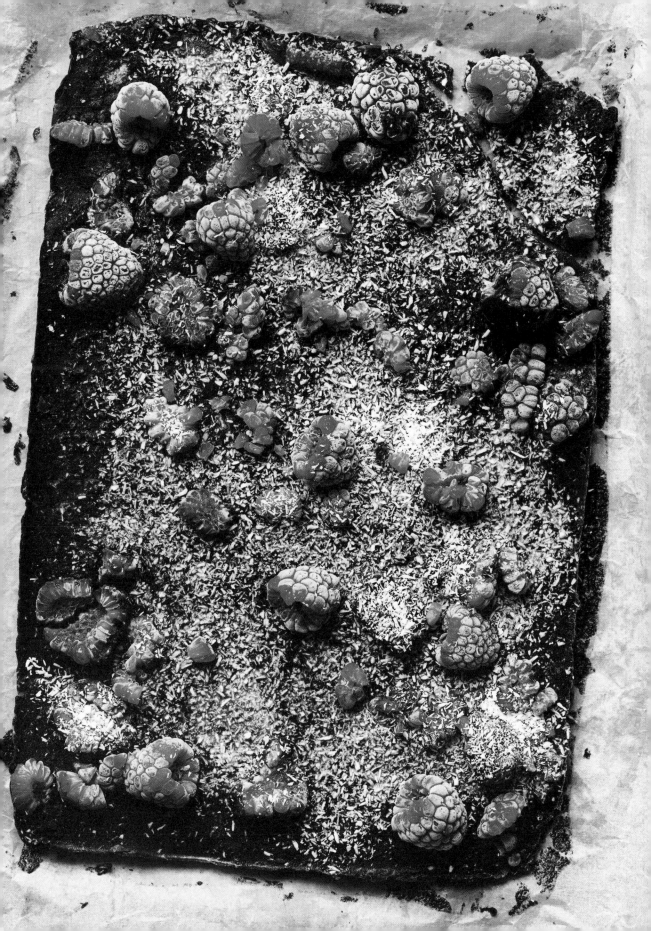

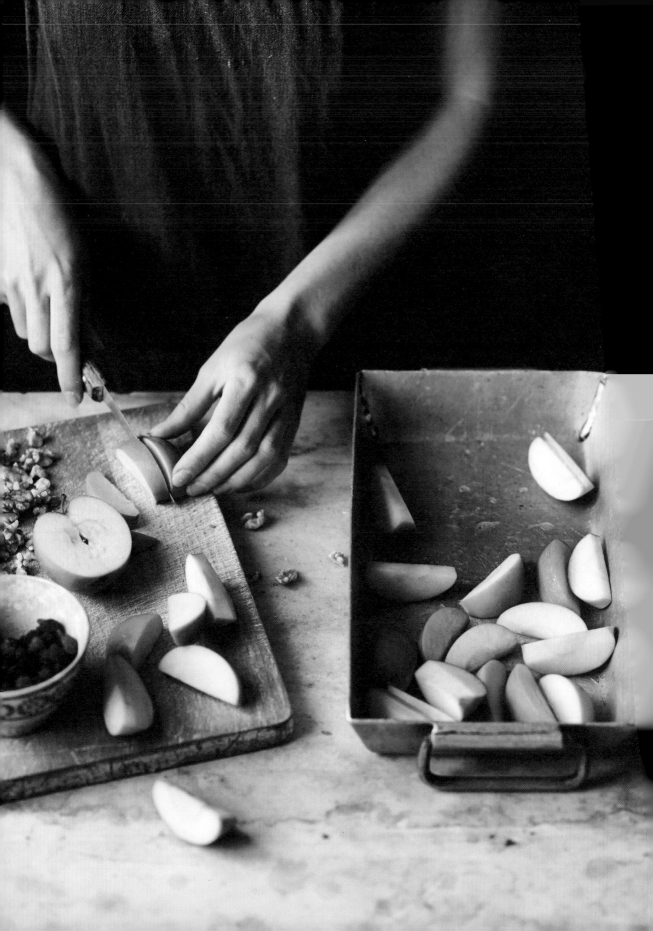

baked apple slices with walnut and cinnamon

I love this easy-to-make and delicious pudding – even more so as it is incredibly nutritious. Apples are a great source of prebiotics and walnuts are rich in healthy fats and fibre, which our gut bacteria love!

Serves 4

2 Tbsp coconut oil (see Tip), melted

4 large apples, cored and cut into wedges

handful of sultanas (golden raisins)

2 tsp ground cinnamon

2 Tbsp chopped walnuts

coconut yoghurt, live natural (plain) yoghurt or organic Greek yoghurt, to serve

df gf vg

1 / Preheat the oven to 160°C (325°F/gas 3).

2 / Brush the base of a baking dish or tin (pan) with a little of the melted coconut oil. Arrange the apple wedges in the baking dish, pour over the remaining coconut oil, scatter with the sultanas and sprinkle over the cinnamon. Bake in the oven for 15 minutes.

3 / Remove from the oven and sprinkle over the chopped walnuts. Increase the oven temperature to 180°C (350°F/gas 4) and return the dish to the oven to bake for a further 8–10 minutes until starting to brown.

4 / Serve with coconut yoghurt, live natural (plain) yoghurt or Greek yoghurt.

tips
Make your own Coconut Oil to use in this recipe (see page 200).

chocolate cups

Vegan, gluten-free and dairy-free! The coconut cream makes these ultra-creamy, and they are just as delicious as they are or topped with peanut butter. If you prefer a sweeter taste or are preparing these for children, do add a little more maple syrup to taste.

Makes 10 cups

100g (3½oz/scant ½ cup) coconut oil (see Tip), melted

3 Tbsp unsweetened cocoa powder or raw cacao powder

2 Tbsp coconut cream

2 Tbsp maple syrup

peanut butter, for topping (optional)

df gf vg

1 / Mix the coconut oil and cocoa powder together in a bowl, then add the coconut cream and maple syrup and mix until it resembles a smooth lump-free paste, adding extra maple syrup to taste, if required.

2 / Place 10 mini paper cupcake cases on a plate and line the bottom of each case with a layer of the chocolate mixture. Pop into the freezer for 5–7 minutes, until the chocolate is firm to the touch.

3 / Remove from the freezer, spread a little peanut butter (if using) on top of each chocolate cup, and place in the fridge for 40 minutes to set.

4 / Serve straight from the fridge. These will keep for 3 days in an airtight container in the fridge.

tips

If you choose to eat these topped with a nut butter, you can use any type you have to hand. They also taste great with hazelnut butter or almond butter.

Make your own Coconut Oil to use in this recipe (see page 200).

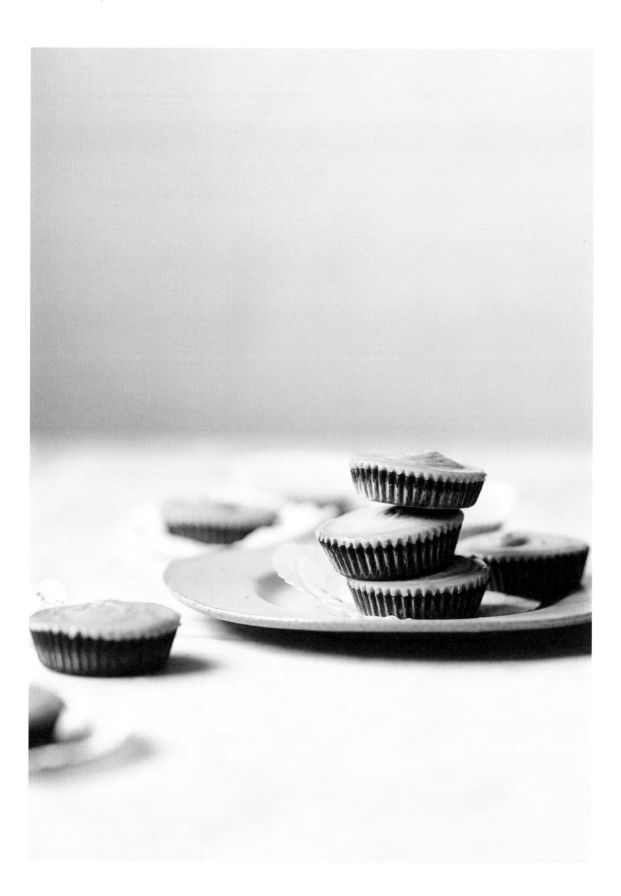

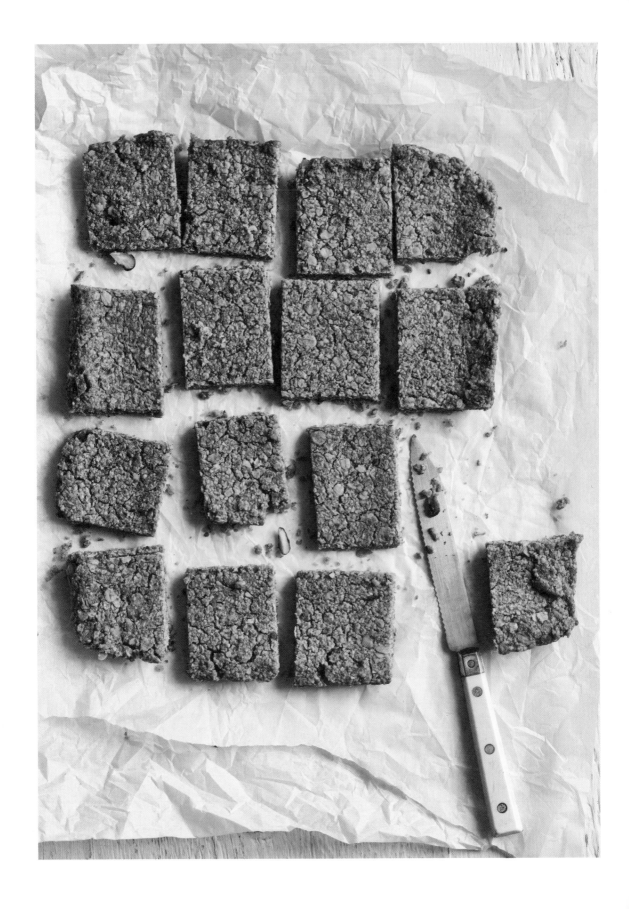

honey flapjack bites

I sweeten these flapjack bites with a little honey and Medjool dates. Medjool dates are a healthy substitute for white refined sugar in pudding recipes, as they are nutritious, being a good source of magnesium, copper, potassium, antioxidants and fibre.

Makes 16 flapjacks

5 Medjool dates

1 tsp ground cinnamon

1 Tbsp honey

1 Tbsp mixed nuts

80g (3oz/⅓ cup) butter, melted

125g (4½oz/1¼ cups) gluten-free rolled oats (oatmeal/old-fashioned oats), gluten-free if necessary

1 / Preheat the oven to 180°C (350°F/gas 4) and line a lipped baking sheet with baking paper.

2 / Put the dates into a bowl and cover with boiling water – ensure they are submerged. Leave for 8–10 minutes, or until softened, then drain and remove the pits.

3 / Put the dates, cinnamon, honey, nuts and butter into a food processor and blitz until smooth. Add the oats and pulse 5–6 times, ensuring you don't over-mix, as you want to retain the texture of the oats.

4 / Pour the mixture onto the prepared baking sheet and press it down well with your hands. Bake in the oven for 12–15 minutes, or until golden.

5 / Remove from the oven and firmly press the mixture down with a spoon – this will prevent the flapjacks from crumbling once they have cooled. Set aside to cool, then transfer to the fridge for 1–1½ hours.

6 / Remove from the fridge and cut into squares.

options
For a dairy-free option, replace the butter with a dairy-free spread.

tips
If the mixture is too crumbly, keep it in the fridge for a couple of hours to firm up.

Leave out the honey if you are looking to reduce your refined sugar intake, and experiment instead by adding finely chopped apple and a handful of sultanas (golden raisins).

almond butter cookies

Almond butter is a good source of protein, healthy monounsaturated fat, fibre, magnesium and vitamin E. In fact, almond butter contains nearly three times as much vitamin E, twice as much iron and seven times more calcium than peanut butter.

Makes 15 cookies

120g (4½oz/generous ½ cup) almond butter

125ml (4fl oz/½ cup) maple syrup

3 Tbsp coconut oil (see Tip)

½ tsp sea salt (kosher salt)

90g (3oz/⅔ cup) almonds, chopped

130g (4¾oz/1 cup) spelt flour

½ tsp bicarbonate of soda (baking soda)

df vg

1 / Preheat the oven to 180°C (350°F/gas 4) and line a baking sheet with baking paper.

2 / In a large bowl, mix together the almond butter, maple syrup, coconut oil, sea salt and most of the almonds, reserving some to decorate.

3 / Meanwhile, in a separate bowl, combine the spelt flour and bicarbonate of soda, then add to the almond butter mixture, stirring well to combine. Set aside for 5 minutes.

4 / Form the dough into 15 individual balls and arrange on the baking sheet, spacing them well apart. Flatten the balls to about 5mm (¼in) thick and scatter over the reserved chopped almonds. Bake in the oven for 10–12 minutes until golden.

5 / Store in an airtight container for up to 5 days.

options
For a gluten-free option, replace the spelt flour with gluten-free plain (all-purpose) flour.

tips
If, like me, you love almond and would like an even stronger almond taste, try adding 1 tsp almond extract.

Spice it up by adding 1 tsp cinnamon for an extra kick.

Make your own Coconut Oil to use in this recipe (see page 200).

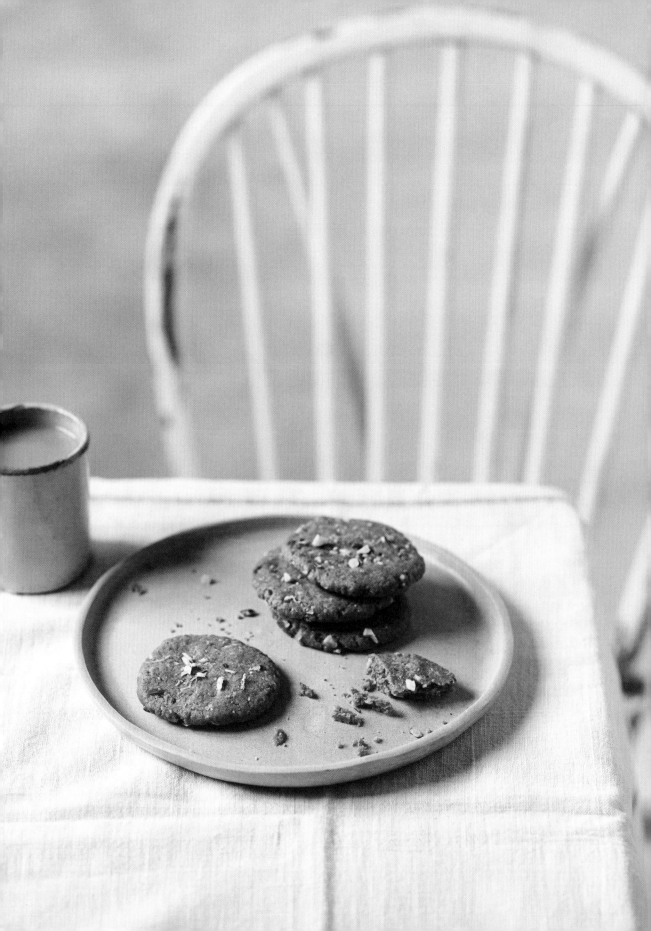

fruit 'n' nut quinoa crumble

I use quinoa in this crumble as it is a great protein source – as are nuts, which are also very good sources of vitamin E, magnesium and selenium. I particularly like to use Brazil nuts, as they are incredibly nutritious and are the richest food source of selenium available. This important mineral plays a vital role in supporting your immune system and promotes immunity by lowering oxidative stress in your body. Nuts also contain anti-inflammatory properties and are high in fibre, which helps you to feel satiated, reduces calorie absorption and promotes gut health

Serves 4

140g (5oz/¾ cup) cooked quinoa

50g (2oz/½ cup) Brazil nuts, roughly chopped

50g (2oz/½ cup) pecans, roughly chopped

50g (2oz/½ cup) walnuts, roughly chopped

30g (1oz/generous ⅓ cup) desiccated (unsweetened dried shredded) coconut

4 Tbsp maple syrup

3 Tbsp coconut oil (see Tip), melted

150g (5½oz/2 cups) frozen raspberries

150g (5½oz/2 cups) frozen blueberries

100g (3½oz/1⅓ cups) frozen blackberries

coconut yoghurt, to serve

df gf vg

1 / Preheat the oven to 180°C (350°F/gas 4).

2 / Put the quinoa, nuts and coconut into a food processor and lightly pulse 2–3 times to combine.

3 / Mix the maple syrup and coconut oil in a bowl, then stir in the nutty quinoa mixture.

4 / Scatter the frozen berries over a baking dish, cover with the crumble mix and bake in the oven for 25 minutes.

5 / Serve with coconut yoghurt.

tips
Make your own Coconut Oil to use in this recipe (see page 200).

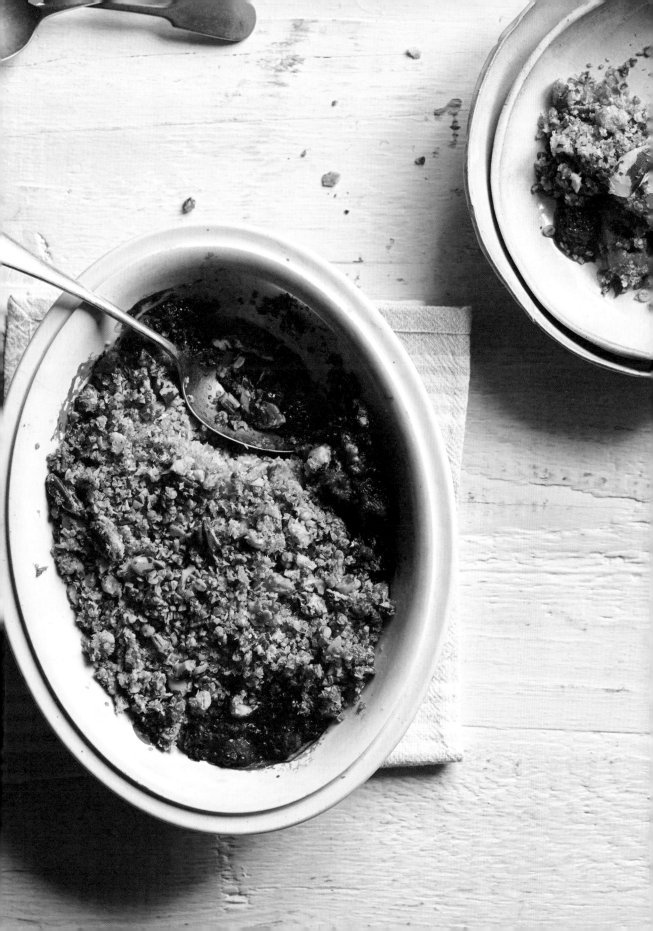

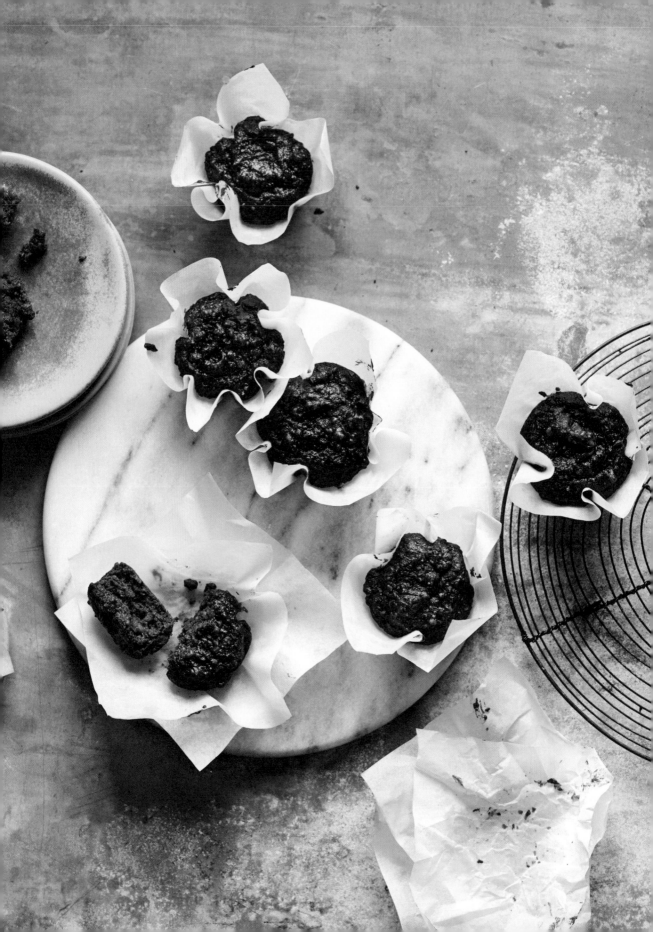

peanut butter bean brownies

I use black beans to replace the flour in these gluten-free, intensely chocolatey, delicious treats. Black beans are incredibly nutritious and loaded with fibre, folate and potassium – they pack a powerful protein punch, too.

Makes 20

1 x 250g (8oz) can black beans, drained and rinsed

150g (5½oz/1½ cups) gluten-free rolled oats (oatmeal/old-fashioned oats)

40g (1½oz/generous ⅓ cup) raw cacao powder

2 tsp gluten-free baking powder

4 eggs

1 Tbsp maple syrup

4 Tbsp peanut butter

2 tsp vanilla extract

225ml (7½fl oz/scant 1 cup) nut milk or oat milk, or more as needed

2 ripe bananas

15 Medjool dates, pitted

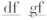

1 / Preheat the oven to 180°C (350°F/gas 4).

2 / Arrange 20 paper cupcake cases in a couple of cupcake or muffin tins (pans).

3 / Place all the ingredients in a food processor or blender and process to a smooth texture. Add more oat or nut milk, if needed.

4 / Pour the mixture into the individual paper cases. Bake in the oven for 12–15 minutes, or until the tops spring back when lightly pressed with a finger. Remove from the oven and place on a wire rack to cool.

options
For a vegan option, replace the eggs with 1 Tbsp chia seeds.

tips
If you don't have raw cacao powder to hand, you can use unsweetened cocoa powder.

Try experimenting with this recipe: add 2 Tbsp chopped walnuts and 2 Tbsp freshly brewed coffee for a coffee and walnut brownie. Alternatively, try adding ½ tsp mint extract for a chocolate mint brownie. Both of these options are absolutely delicious.

index

references

Part 1

Chapter 1

1. CDC 2020, viewed 24 May 2020, www.cdc.gov [https://www.cdc.gov/flu/pandemic-resources/2009-h1n1-pandemic.html]

2. Autoimmune Diseases Coordinating Committee. Progress in Autoimmune Diseases Research: Report to Congress. US Department of Health and Human Services (2005); Rose NR, Mackay IR. Prospectus: the road to autoimmune disease. In: Rose NR, Mackay IR, editors. The Autoimmune Diseases. 4th ed. St. Louis, MO: Academic Press (2006) xix-xxv

3. EAACI 2020, viewed 24 May 2020, www.eaaci.org [https://www.eaaci.org/documents/EAACI_Advocacy_Manifesto.pdf]

4. NHS, 2020, viewed 25th May 2020 [https://www.nhs.uk/conditions/allergies/]

5. WHO 2020, viewed 25 May 2020, www.who.int [https://www.who.int/news-room/fact-sheets/detail/the-top-10-causes-of-death]

6. FSA 2017, viewed 25 May 2020, www.food.gov.uk [https://www.food.gov.uk/sites/default/files/media/document/fsa170306.pdf]

7. Turner PJ, G. M. Increase in anaphylaxis-related hospitalizations but no increase in fatalities: An analysis of United Kingdom national anaphylaxis data, 1992-2012. 2015. J Allergy Clin Immunol, 135(4), 956-963

8. Allergy UK 2020, viewed 25 May 2020, www.allergyuk.org [https://www.allergyuk.org/information-and-advice/statistics]

9. Pawankar R, C. G. 2013. The World Allergy Association (WAO) White Book on Allergy: Update 2013

10. WHO, 2020, viewed 25th May 2020 [https://www.who.int/news-room/fact-sheets/detail/asthma]

11. Asthma UK 2020, viewed 25 May 2020, www.asthma.org.uk [https://www.asthma.org.uk/about/media/facts-and-statistics/]

Chapter 2

12. Alberts, B. et al. Molecular Biology of the Cell, 4th edn. 2002. New York: Garland Science

13. Nicholson, L. 'The immune system'. Essays Biochem. 2016 Oct 31; 60(3): pp.275-301

14. Castellino, F., Galli, G., Del Giudice, G. and Rappuoli, R. 'Generating memory with vaccination'. Eur. J. Immunol. 2009. 39: pp.2100-2105

15. Turner, R. 'Rhinovirus: More than Just a Common Cold Virus'. The Journal of Infectious Diseases, Volume 195, Issue 6, 15 March 2007, pp.765-766

16. Brodin, P. et al. 'Variation in the human immune system is largely driven by non-heritable influences'. 2015. Cell. Volume 160, issue 1-2, pp.37-47

Chapter 3

17. Ubeda, F. and Jansen, V. The evolution of sex-specific virulence in infectious diseases, 2016

18. CDC 2020, viewed 24 May 2020, www.cdc.gov [https://www.cdc.gov/nchs/nvss/vsrr/covid_weekly/index.htm#Race_Hispanic-]

19. Klein, S. L. 'Sex influences immune response to viruses, and efficacy of prophylaxis and treatment for viral diseases'. 2012. Bioessays 34, pp.1050-1059;

    Fish, E. N. 'The X-files in immunity: sex-based differences predispose immune responses'. 2008. Nat. Rev. 8, pp.737-744

20. JRDF 2020, viewed 25 May 2020, www.jdrf.org.uk [https://jdrf.org.uk/news/research-first-could-help-four-million-with-autoimmune-conditions-in-the-uk/]

21. Vojdani, A. et al. Autoimmune Dis. Environmental Triggers and Autoimmunity. 2014; 2014: 798029

22. Ghosh, M., Rodriguez-Garcia, M., Wira, C. 'The Immune System in Menopause: Pros and Cons of Hormone Therapy'. J Steroid Biochem Mol Biol. 2014 Jul; 142:171-5

23. Alduraywish SA, et al. The march from early life food sensitization to allergic disease: a systematic review and meta-analyses of birth cohort studies. Allergy. 2016; 71:77-89

24. CDC, 2020, viewed 24th May 2020 [https://www.cdc.gov/healthyschools/foodallergies/index.htm]

25. Hill, D. and Spergel, J. 'The Atopic March: critical evidence and clinical relevance'. Ann Allergy Asthma Immunol. 2018 Feb; 120(2): pp.131-137

26. Bantz, S.K. et al. 'The Atopic March: Progression from Atopic Dermatitis to Allergic Rhinitis and Asthma'. J Clin Cell Immunol. 2014 Apr; 5(2): 202

27. Mirzakhanni, H. et al. 'Vitamin D and the development of allergic disease: how important is it?' Clin Exp Allergy. 2015 Jan; 45(1):114-125

28. Ozdemir, O. et al. 'Food intolerances and esophagitis in childhood'. 2009. Dig Dis Sci. 2009 Jan;54(1):8-14

29. BDA, 2015, viewed 24th May 2020 [https://www.bda.uk.com/resource/food-allergy-food-intolerance.html]

30. Rona, R.J. et al. 'The prevalence of food allergy: a meta-analysis'. J Allergy Clin Immunol. 2007;120:638-46

31. Perkin et al. 'Randomised trial of introduction of allergenic foods in breast fed infants'. NEJM 2016; 374: 1733-1743

32. Sampson, H.A. et al. 'Food allergy: A practice parameter update-2014'. J Allergy Clin Immunol 2014

33. Maurer, M. 'Cold urticaria'. UpToDate. Updated Apr 2020;

    Stepaniuk, P. et al, Vostretsova, K., Kanani, A. 'Review of cold-induced urticaria characteristics, diagnosis and management in a Western Canadian allergy practice'. Allergy Asthma Clin Immunol. 2018; 14: 85: Published 18 Dec 2018

Chapter 4

34. Lederberg, J., McCray, A.T. "Ome sweet 'omics - a genealogical treasury of words'. Scientist. 2001;15(7):8-8

35. Clarke, G., O'Toole, P.W., Dinan, T.G., Cryan, J.F. 'Characterizing the gut microbiome: role in brain-gut function'. In: Coppola, G., ed. The OMICS: Applications in Neuroscience. Oxford, UK: Oxford University Press; 2014; 265-287;

    Weinstock, G.M. 'Genomic approaches to studying the human microbiota'. Nature. 2012; 489; 250-256

36. Morgan, X.C., Segata, N., Huttenhower, C. 'Biodiversity and functional genomics in the human microbiome'. Trends Genet. 2013; 29; 51-58;

    Human Microbiome Project Consortium. 'Structure, function and diversity of the healthy human microbiome'. Nature. 2012; 486; 207-214

37. Clarke, G. 'Minireview: Gut Microbiota: The Neglected Endocrine Organ'. Mol Endocrinol. 2014 Aug; 28(8): 1221-1238

38. Appleton, J. 'The Gut-Brain Axis: Influence of Microbiota on Mood and Mental Health'. Integr Med (Encinitas). 2018 Aug; 17(4): 28-32

39. Shao, Y. et al. 'Stunted microbiota and opportunistic pathogen colonization in caesarean-section birth'. 2019. Nature volume 574, pp.117-121

40. Marrs, T. 'Is there an association between microbial exposure and food allergy? A systematic review'. Pediatr Allergy Immunol (2013). 24(4): 311-20.e8

41. Fellows, R. et al. 'Microbiota derived short chain fatty acids promote histone crotonylation in the colon through histone deacetylases'. Nature Communications, 2018; 9 (1)

42. Dethlefsen, L. et al. 'The pervasive effects of an antibiotic on the human gut microbiota, as revealed by deep 16s rRNA sequencing'. 2008. PLoS Biol. 2008 Nov 18; 6(11):e280

43. Menees, S., Chey, W. 'The gut microbiome and irritable bowel syndrome'. F1000Res. 2018; 7

44. Weaver, K.R., Melkus, G.D., Henderson, W.A. 'Irritable Bowel Syndrome'. Am J Nurs. 2017;117:48–55

Part 2

Chapter 5
45. Queipo-Ortuño, M. et al. 'Influence of red wine polyphenols and ethanol on the gut microbiota ecology and biochemical biomarkers'. American Journal of Clinical Nutrition, 2012. 95(6), 1323–1334

46. Gibson, G. et al. 'Dietary prebiotics: Current status and new definition'. Food Sci. Technol. Bull. Funct. Foods. 2010; 7:1–19

47. Goldenberg, J.Z. 'Probiotics for the prevention of Clostridium difficle-associated diarrhea in adults and children'. May 2013. Cochrane Database Syst Rev. 5:CD006095

Chapter 6
48. Singh, R. et al. 'Influence of diet on the gut microbiome and implications for human health'. Journal of Translational Medicien 15. Article number 73 (2017)

49. Roblee, M. et al. 'Saturated fatty acids engage in IRE1a-dependent pathway to activate the NLRP3 Inflammasome in Myeloid Cells'. Cell Reports. Vol 14, issue 11. March 22, 2016. pp.2611–2623

50. Hooper, L. et al. 'Reduction in saturated fat intake for cardiovascular disease'. Cochrane Systematic Review – Intervention Version, published 10 June 2015. [https://doi.org/10.1002/14651858.CD011737]

51. British Nutrition Foundation 2020, viewed 28 May 2020, www.nutrition.org.uk [https://www.nutrition.org.uk/nutritionscience/nutrients-food-and-ingredients/fat.html?start=4]

52. American Heart Association 2020, viewed 12 June 2020, [https://www.heart.org/en/healthy-living/healthy-eating/eat-smart/fats/monounsaturated-fats]

53. Burdge, G. 'Metabolism of alpha-linolenic acid in humans'. Prostglandins Leukot Essent Fatty Acids. 2006 Sep; 75(3):161–8;

Brenna, T.J. 'Efficiency of conversion of alpha-linolenic acid to long chain n-3 fatty acids in man'. 2002. Curr Opin Nutr Metab Care. 5(2) 127–32;

Plourde, M. and Cunnane, S. 'Extremely limited synthesis of long chain polyunsaturates in adults: implication for their dietary essentiality and use as supplements'. 2007. Appl Physiol Nutr. Metab. 32(4):619–34

54. Gregersen, S. et al. 'Inflammatory and Oxidative Stress Responses to High-Carbohydrate and High-Fat Meals in Healthy Humans'. 2012. Journal of Nutrition and Metabolism. Vol 2012. Article ID 238056 [https://doi.org/10.1155/2012/238056]

55. Magnusson, K. et al. 'Relationships between Diet-Related Changes in the Gut Microbiome and Cognitive Flexibility'. Neuroscience. 6 Aug 2015;300:128–40

56. Sun, Q., Li, J., Gao, F. 'New insights into insulin: The anti-inflammatory effect and its clinical relevance'. World Journal of Diabetes. Baishideng Publishing Group Inc. 5(2), 89

57. Sherry, C. et al. 'Sickness behavior induced by endotoxin can be mitigated by the dietary soluble fiber, pectin, through up-regulation of IL-4 and Th2 polarization'. Brain Behav Immun. 2010 May; 24(4): 631–640

58. Sonnenbury et al. 'Diet-induced extinctions in the gut microbiota compound over generations'. 2016. Nature volume 529, pp.212–215

59. Bacha et al. 'Nutraceutical, Anti-Inflammatory, and Immune Modulatory Effects of □-Glucan Isolated from Yeast'. 2017. Biomed Res Int. 2017; 2017: 8972678

60. Li, P. et al. 'Amino acids and immune function'. Br J Nutr. 2007 Aug; 98(2):237–52

61. Bauer, J. et al. 'Evidence-based Recommendations for Optimal Dietary Protein Intake in Older People: A Position Paper From the PROT-AGE Study Group'. J Am Med Dir Assoc. Aug 2013; 14(8):542–59

Chapter 7
62. Huang, Z. et al. 'Role of vitamin A in the Immune System'. J Clin Med. 2018 Sep; 7(9): 258

63. NIH 2020, viewed 12 June 2020 [https://ods.od.nih.gov/factsheets/VitaminA-HealthProfessional/]

64. Hong, J.M. et al. 'Vitamin C is taken up by human T cells via sodium-dependent vitamin C transporter 2 (SVCT2) and exerts inhibitory effects on the activation of these cells in vitro'. Anat Cell Biol. 2016; 49(2):88–98

65. Hemilä, H. and Chalker, E. 'Vitamin C for treating and preventing the common cold'. Cochrane Database Syst Rev. 2013 Jan 31;(1):CD000980. DOI: 10.1002/14651858.CD000980.pub4

66. Rode von Essen, M. 'Vitamin D controls T cell antigen receptor signaling and activation of human T cells'. 2010. Nature Immunology, volume 11, pp.344–349

67. Yang, C. et al. 'The Implication of Vitamin D and Autoimmunity: a Comprehensive Review'. Clin Rev Allergy Immunol. 2013 Oct; 45(2): 217–226

68. Mawer et al. 'The distribution and storage of vitamin D and its metabolites in human tissues'. Clin Sci.1972;42(3):413–431;

Abbas, M.A. 'Physiological functions of Vitamin D in adipose tissue'. J Steroid Biochem Mol Biol. 2017; 165(Pt B):369–381

69. National Institutes of Health (2020), viewed 30th June 2020. https://ods.od.nih.gov/factsheets/VitaminE-Consumer/

70. Prasad, A.S. 'Zinc in human health: effect of zinc on immune cells'. Mol Med. 2008;14(5-6):353–357

71. Bonaventura, P. et al. 'Zinc and its role in immunity and inflammation'. Autoimmun Rev. 2015;14(4):277–285

72. Ibs, K. et al. 'Diet and Human Immune Function'. Totowa, New Jersey: Human Press Inc.; 2004:241–259

73. Roy, M. et al. 'Supplementation with selenium and human immune cell functions. I. Effect on lymphocyte proliferation and interleukin 2 receptor expression'. Biol Trace Elem Res. 1994;41(1-2):103–114;

Broome, C.S., McArdle, F., Kyle, J.A. et al. 'An increase in selenium intake improves immune function and poliovirus handling in adults with marginal selenium status'. Am J Clin Nutr. 2004;80(1):154–162

74. Hoffmann, P.R. and Berry, M.J. 'The influence of selenium on immune responses'. Mol Nutr Food Res. 2008;52(11):1273–1280

75. Chandra, R. 'Effect of vitamin and trace element supplementation on immune responses and infection in elderly subjects'. 1992. Lancet, vol 340; pp.1124–7

76. Hamishehkar, H. et al. 'Vitamins are they safe?' Adv Pharm Bull. 2016 Dec; 6(4): 467–477

Chapter 8
77. Remely, M. et al. 'Increased gut microbiota diversity and abundance of Faecalibacterium prausnitzii and Akkermansia after fasting: a pilot study'. Wien Klin Wochenschr. 2015; 127(9-10): 394–398

78. Özkul, C., Yalınay, M. and Karakan, T. 'Islamic fasting leads to an increased abundance of Akkermansia muciniphila and Bacteroides fragilis group: A preliminary study on intermittent fasting'. 2019.Turk J Gastroenterol. 2019 Dec; 30(12): 1030–1035

79. Özkul, C., Yalınay, M. and Karakan, T. 'Structural Changes in Gut Microbiome after Ramadan Fasting: A Pilot Study'. Benef Microbes. 2020 May 11; 11(3): 227–233

80. Cheng, C. et al. 'Prolonged fasting reduces IGF-1/PKA to promote hematopoietic-stem-cell-based regeneration and reverse immunosuppression'. 2014. Cell Stem. Volume 14, issue 6, 810-823;

    Longo, V. The Longevity Diet. 2018. Michael Joseph

81. Choi, Y. et al. 'Nutrition and fasting mimicking diets in the prevention and treatment of autoimmune diseases and immunosenescence'. 2017. Mol Cell Endocrinol. 2017 Nov 5; 455: 4–12

Chapter 9

82. De Heredia, F.P., Gomez-Martinez, S. and Marcos, A. 'Chronic and degenerative diseases: Obesity, inflammation and the immune system'. Proceedings of the Nutrition Society. Cambridge University Press. pp.332–338

83. Viloria, M. et al. 'Effect of moderate exercise on IgA levels and lymphocyte count in mouse intestine'. Immunol Invest. 2011; 40:640–56

84. Matsumoto, M. et al. 'Voluntary running exercise alters microbiota composition and increases n-butyrate concentration in rat cecum'. 2008. Bioscience, Biotechnology and Biochemistry. Volume 72, 2008 – Issue 2

85. Singh, R, et al. 'Influence of diet on the gut microbiome and implications for human health'. J Transl Med. 2017; 15: 73.

86. Nieman et al. 'Immune response to a 30 minute walk'. Medicine and Science in Sports and Exercise. 01 Jan 2005, 37(1):57–62

87. Simpson, R. et al. 'Can Exercise Affect Immune Function to Increase Susceptibility to Infection?' Exerc Immunol Rev, 2020

88. NHS 2020, viewed 28 May 2020 [https://www.nhs.uk/live-well/exercise/]

89. Barrett, B. et al. 'Meditation or exercise for preventing acute respiratory infection'. The Annals of Family Medicine. Vol.10, Issue 4. July/August 2012

Chapter 10

90. Kiecolt-Glaser, J. K., Glaser, R. (1993). 'Mind and immunity'. In: D. Goleman & J. Gurin, (Eds.) Mind/Body Medicine (pp. 39-59). New York: Consumer Reports

91. Segerstrom, S. C. and Miller, G. E. (2004). 'Psychological Stress and the Human Immune System: A Meta-Analytic Study of 30 Years of Inquiry'. Psychological Bulletin, Vol. 130, No. 4.

92. Schnall et al. 'Social support and the perception of geographical slant'. Journal of Experimental Social Psychology. Volume 44, Issue 5, September 2008, pp.1246–1255

93. Karl, J.P. et al. 'Effect of psychological, environmental and physical stressors on the gut microbiota'. Front Microbiol. 2018; 9: 2013

94. Mackos, A.R., Maltz, R., Bailey, M.T. (2017). 'The role of the commensal microbiota in adaptive and maladaptive stressor-induced immunomodulation.' Horm. Behav. 88 70–78

95. Mawdsley, J.E., Rampton, D.S. (2005). 'Psychological stress in IBD: new insights into pathogenic and therapeutic implications'. Gut 54 1481–1491;

    Konturek, P.C., Brzozowski, T., Konturek, S.J. (2011). 'Stress and the gut: pathophysiology, clinical consequences, diagnostic approach and treatment options'. J. Physiol. Pharmacol. 62 591–599

96. Bailey, M. et al. 'Exposure to a Social Stressor Alters the Structure of the Intestinal Microbiota: Implications for Stressor-Induced Immunomodulation'. Brain Behav Immun. 2011 Mar;25(3):397–407

97. Michalsen, A. et al. 'Rapid Stress Reduction and Anxiolysis Among Distressed Women as a Consequence of a Three-Month Intensive Yoga Program'. Med Sci Monit. 2005 Dec;11(12):555–561

98. Smith, C. et al. 'A Randomised Comparative Trial of Yoga and Relaxation to Reduce Stress and Anxiety'. Complement Ther Med. 2007 Jun;15(2):77–83

99. Orme-Johnson and Barnes, V. 'Effects of the Transcendental Meditation Technique on Trait Anxiety: A Meta-Analysis of Randomized Controlled Trials'. Altern Complement Med. 2014 May; 20(5):330–41

100. Margarey, C. 'Meditation and Health'. Darshan magazine SYDA Foundation, NY 12779, USA

101. Gu, J. et al. 'How do mindfulness-based cognitive therapy and mindfulness-based stress reduction improve mental health and wellbeing? A systematic review and meta-analysis of mediation studies'. Clinical Psychology Review. Volume 37, April 2015, 1–12

Chapter 11

102. CMO de Almeida, 2016; Opp 2015; Opp, M.R. and Krueger, J.M. 'Sleep and immunity: a growing field with clinical impact'. Brain Behav Immun 2015;47:1–3

103. Born, J. et al. 'Effects of sleep and circadian rhythm on human circulating immune cells'. J Immunol 1997;158:4454–64

104. Fondell, E., Axelsson, J., Franck, K., Ploner, A., Lekander, M., Balter, K., et al. 'Short natural sleep is associated with higher T cell and lower NK cell activities'. Brain Behav Immun 2011; 25(7):1367–75

105. Massa, J. et al.' Vitamin D and actigraphic sleep outcomes in older community-dwelling men: the MrOS sleep study'. 2015. Sleep. 2015 Feb 1; 38(2):251–7

106. NHS 2020, viewed 1 June 2020 [https://www.nhs.uk/live-well/sleep-and-tiredness/how-to-get-to-sleep/]

107. Bannai, M. et al. 'The effects of glycine on subjective daytime performance in partially sleep-restricted healthy volunteers'. Front Neurol. 2012; 3():61;

    Inagawa, K. et al. 'Subjective effects of glycine ingestion before bedtime on sleep quality'. Sleep Biol Rhythms. 2006;4:75–77;

    Yamadera, W. et al. 'Glycine ingestion improves subjective sleep quality in human volunteers, correlating with polysomnographic changes'. Sleep Biol Rhythms. 2007; 5:126–131

Chapter 12

108. Yang, CY et al. 'The implication of vitamin D and autoimmunity: a comprehensive review'. Clin Rev Allergy Immunol. 2013 Oct; 45(2): 217-226.

109. Thieu, X. et al. 'Intrinsic Photosensitivity Enhances Motility of T Lymphocytes'. Scientific Reports, 2016; 6: 39479

110. Yamamoto, E. and Jørgensen. 'Relationships between Vitamin D, Gut Microbiome, and Systemic Autoimmunity' Front Immunol. 2019; 10: 3141

111. Luthold, R.V. et al. 'Gut microbiota interactions with the immunomodulatory role of vitamin D in normal individuals'. Metabolism. 2017 Apr; 69():76–86;

    Ooi, J.H., Li, Y., Rogers, C.J., Cantorna, M.T. 'Vitamin D regulates the gut microbiome and protects mice from dextran sodium sulfate – induced colitis 1 – 3'. J Nutr. (2013) 143:1679–86

112. Sahota, O. 'Understanding vitamin D deficiency'. Age Ageing. 2014 Sep; 43(5): 589–591;

    Holick, M.F. 'Vitamin D deficiency'. N Engl J Med. 2007;357:266–81

113. Forrest, K. and Stuhldreher. 'Prevalence and Correlates of Vitamin D Deficiency in US Adults'. Nutr Res. 2011 Jan;31(1):48–54

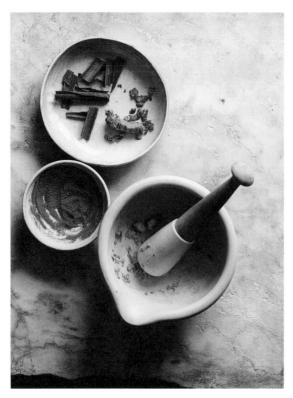
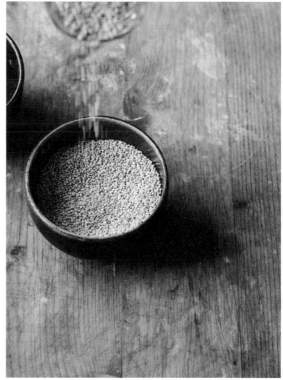

Publishing Director: Sarah Lavelle
Senior Commissioning Editor: Céline Hughes
Designer: Alicia House
Photographer: Steven Joyce
Food Stylist: Kitty Coles
Prop Stylist: Louie Waller
Head of Production: Stephen Lang
Production Controller: Katie Jarvis

Published in 2020 by Quadrille,
an imprint of Hardie Grant Publishing

Quadrille
52–54 Southwark Street
London SE1 1UN
quadrille.com

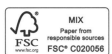

Cataloguing in Publication Data: a catalogue record
for this book is available from the British Library.

Text © Kate Llewellyn-Waters 2020
Photography © Steven Joyce
Design and layouts © Quadrille 2020

ISBN 978 1 78713 679 3

Printed in China